Eli
The Boy Who Hated to Write
Understanding Dysgraphia

Regina G. Richards
Eli I. Richards

Foreword by
Richard D. Lavoie

RET Center Press
Riverside CA
2nd Edition
2008

Eli

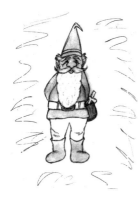

ISBN 0-9661353-6-9

The Boy Who Hated to Write

Dedicated to the memory of Dovid M. Richards

- ◆   *You're forever in our hearts*
- ◆   *You'd be so very proud of Eli*

A favorite quote:

"We must not, in trying to think about how we can make a big difference, ignore the small daily differences we can make which, over time, add up to big differences that we often cannot foresee."

--Marian Wright
Edelman

Contents

Foreword

Did you ever have a job where there was one solitary task that you abhorred or dreaded? Perhaps it was a monthly accounting report or an annual inventory project. You constantly dreaded the day that your superior entered your office to announce that it was time to approach this distasteful and fear-filled activity. You were anxious, frightened and disheartened.

This is the way that Eli Richards – and every child who struggles with dysgraphia – felt each time he heard a teacher say the dreaded words, "Everyone take out a piece of paper…I want you to write a composition…"

Eli is a bright student with an extensive repertoire of interests and talents. He has a rich and vibrant vocabulary and an impressive fund of background information and facts. He is wonderfully creative and has earned the respect and affection of all who know him because of his innovative view of life.

But he couldn't write. Every aspect of the writing process – handwriting, note taking, spelling, syntax, semantics, word choice, etc. – was a mystery for him. His fluency and fluidity with language came to a frightening and screeching halt whenever he sat in front of a blank piece of paper with a pen in hand. As he progressed through the grades, composition skills became increasingly important…and increasingly frustrating and frightening.

But Eli's story is not merely a tale of failure and struggle. It is also a story of support, faith and small victories. Eli's school life had detractors and demons…but he also had defenders and champions. As I read of Eli's struggles, I was reminded that – as in the fairy tales – one caring, devoted adult can save the life of a child.

Dysgraphia is among the least understood aspects of learning disorders. This complex problem has a confusing collection of symptoms and manifestations. These children wrestle daily with a Gordian knot of attention problems, memory difficulties, language deficiencies and idiosyncratic thought processes. Often, the professionals in the child's life will deal with the individual symptoms of Dysgraphia, but they fail to understand (or remediate) the disorder in its entirety. They assist with the symptoms without confronting the problem in any way. As a result, their interventions are often unsuccessful and the child's frustrations become more profound.

Eli – The Boy Who Couldn't Write puts a human face on this puzzling disorder. In a charming and insightful narrative, Eli tells of his daily frustrations and his creative attempts to avoid – and later, self-remediate – his writing problems. You feel as if you are sitting next to Eli in the classroom as he faces his daily challenges.

Eli's story of fear, frustration and failure enables the reader to gain a genuine understanding of the problems that Eli confronted daily. But the book is not only about struggles…it also offers solutions. At the conclusion of Eli's narrative…the calvary arrives offering practical advice for how we can assist the dysgraphic child in the classroom and at home.

Eli's mother, Regina, has come to be recognized as one of the nation's foremost experts on this puzzling disorder. She provides a detailed but understandable list of dysgraphia's symptoms and etiology. As you read her outline, you will come to recognize the dysgraphic students in your own classroom. Beyond merely identifying the disorder, Regina offers field-tested strategies and approaches to use with the child. By combining her unparalleled experiences as a teacher, consultant and researcher with her experiences as "Eli's Mom", she is able to approach this task with the mind of a professional…and the heart of a parent. An unbeatable combination.

As you read Eli's story, allow his compelling words to solidify your commitment to the children in your life who fight the "writing dragon" daily.

With every good wish,

Richard D. Lavoie
President
Riverview School

Richard D Lavoie, M.A., M.Ed.
Visiting Lecturer, Harvard University
Author, *It's So Much work to Be Your Friend: Helping the Child with Learning Disabilities Find Social Success*, and *The Motivation Breakthrough: 6 Secrets to Turning On the Tuned-Out Child*

Eli

Preface

We wrote this book for one reason: dysgraphia is so frequently misunderstood.

When Eli was in his third year of college, he came home one day claiming, teachers just don't understand! As we discussed what was going on, it was obvious that Eli was indeed correct: his English teacher didn't understand the issues he was dealing with regarding his dysgraphia. He wanted me to write a book to give her. I explained that it would be more efficient to have a book explaining the student's perspective when dealing with writing issues. He was horrified at the idea of "writing a book," but as we discussed the concept of using his Dragon Naturally Speaking (speech to text computer program), and when I promised to be his editor, he warmed to the idea. The result of that discussion was the first edition of *Eli, The Boy Who Hated to Write*. Students, parents and educators loved the simplicity and informative nature of the book.

Far too frequently, students with a processing pattern such as dysgraphia fail to demonstrate what they know because of their interfering struggles to communicate using the written word. Eli and I want to further share his experiences so that others who struggle will know they are not alone, and so they will be a little more comfortable with their differences. At the same time, we want to provide information to help parents and teachers better understand this issue, as well as related issues that affect written efficiency. After all, greater understanding is the first step towards developing an ability to reach out and help others.

This second edition of *Eli, The Boy Who Hated to Write*, provides additional narratives related to Eli's experiences during time periods before and after the 5th grade experiences he discussed in the first Edition. Furthermore, the Commentaries at the end of the book are greatly expanded to provide teachers and parents with additional information.

The Boy Who Hated to Write

The creation of any book begins with ideas. Throughout the years, there have been many people who influenced Eli and helped him to understand his issues. Furthermore a great many people have influenced my ideas, enabling me to grow professionally. Thank you to all of them. Special appreciation goes to Dr. Melvin D. Levine, M.D., co-chairman of All Kinds of Minds and pediatrician at the Clinical Center for the Study of Development and Learning (School of Medicine, University of North Carolina at Chapel Hill). I thank you for being my mentor through your many books, articles, and workshops. Your wonderful emphasis on helping children understand their own strengths and weaknesses encouraged me to guide children along this important pathway.

Particular gratitude is extended to Richard Lavoie, M.A., M.Ed., Visiting Lecturer, Harvard University, and author, *It's So Much Work to Be Your Friend: Helping the Child with Learning Disabilities Find Social Success* and *The Motivation Breakthrough: 6 Secrets to Turning On the Tuned-Out Child.* We thank you for sharing with the educational and parental communities your depth of understanding about the process of learning. Your inspiring books, videos and workshops are always an amazing and thought provoking experience.

We also acknowledge some very special and creative artists who enhanced this publication with their drawings.

- Lynn Craven, a very talented high school art teacher, for his drawing of a boy running down the hall

- Judy Love, a creative educational therapist, for her drawings of the gnome and the dolphin

- Vicky L. Jones, for her creative contributions of the picture of the fort in Eli's room and the cave in the forest

Thank you to all.

Eli

Irv Richards, Eli's dad and my superb husband, spent many hours reading various drafts of this manuscript. We thank you for your time and comments and especially for your unending love and support throughout my many projects. I would be much less without your continuing love, guidance, and partnership.

I recall with fondness and humor the first time Eli sent me an email message signed "173". Not having as much visual-spatial flexibility as Eli, it took me a bit to see the connection. Now Irv and I are very familiar with his signature.

Eli, thanks so much for sharing your experiences and your stories. I loved all the time we spent chatting about these things. Most of all, thanks for being you.

Regina G. Richards

Regina G. Richards, M.A.

2008

Prequel: Checkmarks

I wake up with the bright sun shining through my window into my eyes. It's a Monday morning, which begins like any other day of first grade. I get out of bed, wash, and begin to dress, just as the pictured list on my wall tells me. I select my clothes from the "clean clothes" pile on the floor, and I look at my fort as I get dressed.

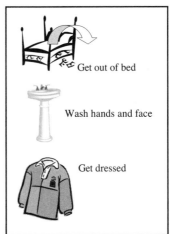

Get out of bed

Wash hands and face

Get dressed

Boy, I really love to build forts. I made this one using a large sturdy white table that used to be a big worktable for my dad. It's higher and much bigger than our dinner table. I decided to put the table in a corner so it's against two walls.

Eli

Mom gave me an old bed sheet. At first, I used scotch tape to hold the sheet around the other two edges of the table. Now I use Velcro. It's so cool to have a fort right here so that I can escape into it any time I want. This is my own private hiding place where I can think and dream; the rest of the world doesn't bother me. So many amazing things happen when I'm inside my fort.

"Hello, Eli," I hear Mom call. "Good morning Son. Come to breakfast."

While I am eating my Cheerios™, I remember that we have reading group after recess today. I begin to think....... maybe, if I disappear into my fort, Mom will get busy with her own work and forget it's a school day.

Nah, the day's not going so good this far – my Cheerios™ aren't even cooperating. My bowl is full, and they keep escaping as I dunk them under the milk. It would just be too good to be true for Mom to forget a school day. But...if I don't take long eating breakfast, then maybe I will have time to crawl into my fort and escape with some great adventure.

After eating breakfast and brushing my teeth, I notice that Mom isn't at the front door yet. Maybe she is forgetting it's a school day. So I quietly scamper to my fort. As usual, Pokey, my little dog, follows me inside. We visit with Peanut, my special friend that only we can see.

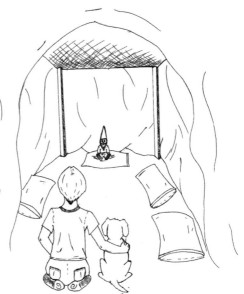

It's fun to talk to Pokey and Peanut. They're both really good listeners! So, I start talking quietly to them.

"Hey Peanut, so much is confusing. Don't

you agree? A while back, I thought I was a pretty good reader. I worked hard with Tutor during the summer to learn all the letters and sounds, and I knew them, mostly. She kept telling me I was doing really well. I thought I was too. So, when we started reading level books at school, I could read just as good as the other kids. We all started out just about the same."

Pokey curled up into my lap and licked my face. Peanut just sat and listened. I continued.

"But, just like everything else, before I knew it, all the other kids were way ahead of me. Bummer! We have to keep practicing each book until we can read it "perfectly" to Teacher. The other kids keep reading book after book. But not me! I'm so far behind— there's no way I'll ever catch up.

It's not fair! It frustrates me to see all my friends pass me up. I sure don't understand why they can do it and I can't.

"These books are only little books. Why can't I read them like the other kids? It used to be fun when we all started reading together. As everyone passes me by, I realize how hard reading is. It's much more work than fun.

Am I stupid? Does my brain just stop working sometimes? I think I know the words, but then when they're all together on a page, they get jumbled. Mom keeps telling me I'm not stupid, but she's just Mom. It's so frustrating. I feel I can't rely on or trust my brain. Peanut, Pokey, what's going on? Being confused like this is a yucky feeling.

"Uh-oh, what's that? Mom's calling me. She didn't forget it's a school day after all. I didn't think she would. Pokey, Peanut, be real quiet. Maybe Mom won't find us."

I hear her coming closer and closer calling, "Eli! Eli! It's time to go to school now. Come on, Eli!"

I remain very quiet. Mom's voice is getting louder, and

now she's yelling, "Eli, you come out right now!" I put my finger to my lips reminding Peanut and Pokey to stay quiet.

We hear Mom even closer now, shouting, "Eli, no more playing around. Get out here, now! Right now!"

I look at Pokey and ask her, "What should I do?" Pokey licks my face. I turn to Peanut and ask the same question, "What should I do? I really don't want to go to school." I think I hear Peanut saying that I had better listen to Mom.

"Eli, if you don't come out right now, you'll go to school in your pajamas," I hear her yell. I guess she forgot that I was already dressed. She must be that mad!

I poke my head out of the fort and see Mom glaring down at me. Pokey notices the tension. As I stand up with her, she licks my face. This makes me laugh. I look at Mom; she's still glaring. I put Pokey down and run to the door. As I get there, I hear her yell, "Don't forget your bag!"

I run back and grin at her as I hug Pokey again and pick up my school bag.

On the way to school, Mom asks what's wrong. Eventually, I tell her that I don't like reading. In fact, I was hoping to miss school today so I won't have to read. She says, "Eli, sometimes you get so caught up thinking about one bad thing in a day that you forget there will be many fun parts in the day as well, like seeing your friends and having recess. Besides, you have your new yo-yo in your backpack. Remember how excited you are about showing it to your friends?"

In class, I'm in my seat thinking that being at school today isn't as bad as I thought. Teacher's in a real happy mood and we're having a lot of fun. Then she makes an announcement, "Class, because today is Jade's birthday, after lunch we'll have a small party with cupcakes". We clap our hands and yell, "Happy birthday Jade".

Eli

After we talk about our weekend adventures, it's craft time. That's not so bad, because Teacher always says nice things about everybody's creation, even mine. When Teacher asks me what I've made, I reply, "It's supposed to be me on my bike with Pokey running along side." She says, "That's great, Eli. It looks like you're having fun with your doggie." I think that's weird, because to me the clay looks like an ugly broken bike with a blob next to it. But it's so nice that she likes it anyway.

While I continue working with my clay, I start thinking about what comes next. After art is recess and then…. ugh, reading time. I sure wish I could read books faster. But, I just can't do it. The words fall out of my head. What's wrong with my brain? This learning stuff is such a big unknown. I just can't understand why some things are so easy, like my puzzles and Legos®. Then some things are so so difficult. When I try something that turns out Ok, it feels really good. It's like "wow". But school is different. When I'm in school, some things are way too hard.

I look up at Teacher's desk and see her pulling out her grade book. She uses this to put a check mark each time one of us kids finish a level book. I saw that page once. Everybody else has lots and lots of check marks. Then by my name, there are only a few. What a disaster.

What in the world can I do to get more check marks by my name? I wonder if I think real hard, I could make Magic put more check marks by my name. If new check marks magically show up on the Eli line, then I will be even with everyone else. I will be as smart as them!

I don't really think Magic can put check marks in Teacher's grade book. I need another plan. But, I'm stuck. I can't think of anything else. I wish Peanut were here. Peanut is Magic. After all, he is a gnome.

I remember when Peanut first came to see me. Way back in kindergarten, things were pretty tough. My pictures and letters were messy. I didn't feel so good about myself.

Eli

I was lonely. I needed someone to talk to and keep me calm. A small gnome came to sit on my shoulder. He began to remind me that I really could do lots of things well. My tiny gnome's name is "Peanut" because he is so small.

I sure wish Peanut was here. He'd help me come up with a good plan. Wait a second. Why is everyone leaving?

What's that I hear? Teacher is talking to me. "Hello Eli. Can't you hear me? Please put away your materials and go to recess."

As I go, I'm still trying to figure out a plan. I have no idea how to magically add check marks in Teacher's grade book. Wait! Where's my yo-yo? Oh yeah —it's in my backpack. Gee. I really wanted to show my friends how I can work it.

On the play yard, I decide to go up to Teacher. "I forgot my yo-yo," I say in my most polite voice. "May I please go back to get it?" "Of course," she says, "but hurry back."

I am inside the classroom and I grab my yo-yo. Turning to run back outside, I notice the grade book sitting open on top of Teacher's desk. Hmmm. Maybe I can peek and see how far behind I really am. I carefully tiptoe over to the desk, looking around to make sure I'm alone.

Wow! The book is open to the page with the list of reading books and all of the check marks. Am I lucky, or what?

While looking at the grade book, my heart sinks right down to my shoes. I really am the lowest person in the class. A sick feeling comes deep in my tummy as I realize how small my line of checkmarks is.

Eli

Suddenly, the room gets really bright, just like a cloud uncovering the sun. Boing! An idea pops right into my head.

After carefully looking around once more and telling my beating heart to beat more quietly, I slowly pick up a pen. Making sure to have the line that goes with my name, I add two check marks. Whew! That was easy. I take a deep breath and think, "Might as well add a few more. Here goes."

Oh look, there's my friend Michael's name. He's not as low as I am but he could probably use a few more marks. I carefully and neatly make two checks in Michael's row. Now Michael is smarter too.

Oh man, my heart is beating so loudly that I'd be surprised if no one heard. Carefully placing the pen back exactly as it was and

Date Beginning		Book #	Ending	
	Day of Week / Date	**1ST WEEK** M T W T F / 1 2 3 4 5	**2ND WEEK** M T W T F / 6 7 8 9 10	**3RD WEEK** M T W T F / 11 12 13 14 15
SUBJECT *Level Books*				
TEACHER *Fall*				
1 *Mario*				
2 *Adelante*	✓✓✓✓✓	✓✓✓	
3 *Maria*				
4 *Benny*	✓✓✓✓✓	✓✓✓✓	✓✓
5 *Michael*				
6 *Friend*	✓✓✓✓✓	✓\\\	
7 *Jose*				
8 *Gary*	✓✓✓✓✓	✓✓	
9 *Anna*				
10 *Mc Coy*	✓✓✓✓✓	✓✓✓✓✓	
11 *Eli*				
12 *Richards*	✓✓✓✓✓✓✓	✓✓	
13 *Jody*				
14 *Riddle*	✓✓✓✓✓	✓✓✓✓	
15 *Sally*				
16 *Smart*	✓✓✓✓✓	✓✓✓✓✓	✓✓
17 *Pete*				
18 *Wonder*	✓✓✓✓✓	✓✓✓	
19 *Jade*				
20 *Zoria*	✓✓✓✓✓	✓	
21				

making sure nothing was moved, I pick up my yo-yo and run back to recess. Oh look, my friends are playing kickball. I guess I didn't need my yo-yo after all.

The bell is ringing. That's our signal recess is finished. It was a great game of kickball.

We're all in our seats inside the classroom now. Teacher announces, "It's reading time" (as if we don't know that!). She picks up her grade book and looks at the list, reminding everyone which book to get. I'm about to grab my usual book but Teacher calls out a different one for me. Oh yeah, how could I forget? I begin to feel a little excited.

Now that I'm smarter, I'll be reading like the others. I'm sure there's no way anyone can discover my little adventure. After all, I only put a few check marks in the book. They are just like the other checkmarks that Teacher made. Besides, I wrote real slowly and made my very neatest marks. I'm sure I'll be able to read my books OK now. Why, then, does my stomach feel like it's in knots?

I see Michael walk up with his book and talk to Teacher, only to go back and get a different book. Teacher looks down at her grade book again. Oh. Oh. She's getting a real funny look on her face. Oh my. I don't feel so good. I'm real worried. Could she possibly know what I did? Or maybe, it's just something else on her mind.

Oh no, now she's looking around the room. She's looking very slowly from row to row, and she has that 'look'. We all know that something is up when Teacher gets that 'look'.

Her gaze pauses at Michael for a few seconds longer than the other kids. Then, she glances back at her grade book. Her head starts moving again. She's moving her head towards my direction. I stare down at my desk, but sneakily peek up. She is looking at me. She keeps looking at me.

Golly gee. It seems that she knows. I know she knows. But how can she? I so carefully and neatly made each check mark.

I become real busy looking for my spot in the reading book. I can't bear to look up. Oh no. I hear her coming toward my desk. I see her shoes. I peek and notice that she is real close and she still has that 'look'. "Class," she says, "practice reading your books silently. I'll be right back."

"Hello, Eli," says Teacher. "Please come with me?"

Oh my gosh! How does she know? My knees are shaking. I can't even respond to her. I try to talk but nothing comes out. Finally, I slowly nod my head up and down.

Teacher takes me to Principal's office and tells me to sit in a chair in the back room. There are no outside windows and no pictures on the walls. I hear her talking quietly to Principal. I think they're laughing, but I'm not sure. No, they can't be *laughing*. Teacher looked terribly mad at me! I know she's furious. Teacher leaves to go back to class. I hear Principal use the phone. Then I hear, "May I please speak to Mrs. Richards?" Her voice gets very very quiet.

Uh-oh! I'm really in for it now. They bothered Mom at work. That's the big no no. I'm not sup- posed to call Mom at work unless it's an emergency. Does this mean that *this* is an emergency? My heart sinks even further, if that's possible.

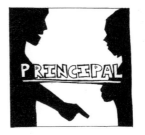

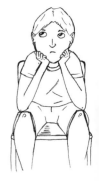

Principal comes into the back room and says, "Hello Eli. You can sit here and wait until your mother arrives. We're going to have a meeting about The Incident. Oh, man. This is surely the end of privileges for the rest of my life! Then Principal hand me a bunch of pages to do. Some are coloring, some are matching, and some are sentences to write.

A long long long time later, Principal comes in and explains that it's now lunchtime. She asks me where my lunch is and I tell her it's in my backpack. It must be at the end of morning. I think, "Yeah! I don't have to read." I've been here so long that I thought it must surely be almost nighttime already. Then Principal says that I will be eating my lunch in the back room today. All alone.

She brings me my lunch. I eat it although I really don't want to. But, there's nothing else to do. I eat very slowly because my stomach is doing big somersaults. Sweat runs down my neck and it's not even hot. Man, oh man, am I ever

Eli

nervous. I wish I could talk to my friend Michael to find out what's going on. He's my very best friend – well, other than Pokey and Peanut. Michael is my very best person friend.

Pretty soon, I hear all the kids outside. Oh heck – my friends already had Jade's birthday party. I hope they saved me a chocolate cupcake. I can't see anything, because I'm in a room with no windows. Usually when I do something wrong, I get 'benched', and I sit on the wooden slab in front of the office during recess. At least then, I can see what all the kids are doing. I can watch them play, and I know what's going on. Now I can't see anybody. This is really awful and boring.

Soon the bell rings, and it gets quiet. This means lunch recess is over, and the kids are back in class. What's going to happen to me? Am I going to have to stay here the rest of my life with these stupid papers?

After another long, long, very long time, Principal comes in and asks me, "Eli, would you like a bathroom break?" I say, "Yes" thinking that at least I'll get to see some different walls for a few minutes.

How humiliating! Principal escorts me to the boys' room and waits outside for me to finish. She escorts me back to the office. What did she think? That I would run home? That I would run to my friends?

When I'm back in my prison room, Principal tells me that Mom will be coming for a meeting in about another hour.

I groan to myself, and sit back, wishing I could be somewhere else.

I sit and play around with the papers Principal gave me. Eventually, after another long time, Mom finally comes for the meeting.

Eli

I'm sure glad that I didn't get any major punishments other than spending that horrible time in the 'prison room'. It turns out that I'm going to begin to work with Teacher three times a week before school. It's a little scary to think about. At least it's before school, and the other kids won't see me.

Prequel: Piano

I think about how amazing it is that I've made it to third grade. Today I'm free and don't have to think about school. It's a school holiday and my friend Michael is coming over to play before we go to our piano lessons.

While waiting for Michael, I build this really cool fort in my living room using a sheet, two blankets, and three big pillows. As I get older, my forts become more elaborate. I arrange this stuff over our sofa and other chairs and create a neat spot in the corner that opens up. We can easily get in and out of the fort.

Pokey and I crawl into the fort. We sit there fooling around and I start thinking of different things.

I remember a few years ago in school when I put those check marks in Teacher's grade book. I sure don't know how she knew that it had been me with such neatly made checkmarks. It sure is confusing how she figured it out. I got in trouble, and that was pretty bad. But afterwards it was interesting. I worked with Teacher before school almost every day and then, during summer, I worked with Teacher's daughter, Tammy.

Tammy is really neat. She's studying to be a teacher at the University. She was already very good at explaining stuff and was just starting her program. She's like my friend, even though she's older. I still work with Tammy after school and sometimes on weekends. She'll finish her program soon and will become a real teacher. I wonder if I will still be able to work with her then.

It's so strange that something that was bad (getting into big-time trouble) turned into something good (learning to read). Mom always tells me to look for something good in a situation even when it starts out real bad. I get more help now and I'm learning to read pretty good. It's still hard and I'm still very slow, but at least I can do it!

My thoughts turn to something else that was really bad but turned into something good. It was maybe a year ago. We had a really fun family dinner and were telling jokes, having a grand time. After dinner, it was my turn to clear the table. When I was done, Mom helped me with my homework, and then I finally got to go back to my room. My room was dark, because the light wasn't on. Before I could even turn on the switch, my closet opened and someone yelled, "BOOOO!"

I was so scared. I'm not sure exactly what I did, except scream really loud. Mom and Dad were both there by my door as I ran out of my room and fell into their arms. Mom said I was shaking like a leaf. Well, of course, I was terrified.

It turns out that Dov was hiding in my closet the whole time since dinner. He was the one who yelled "booo" when I came in the room. It was so unexpected that I didn't even recognize my own brother's voice.

Eli

After I calmed down, I looked at Dov. He was so upset. He was sorry for scaring me so badly. Mom said he didn't think about the consequences before acting. To show me how sorry he was, he gave me one of his favorite toys: a GI Joe.

That's what I mean that something good came after something bad. I was really scared, but then Dov was so nice to me. It felt good that he was nice. He likes to tease me – I guess that's because he's my older brother. Besides, he's good at everything and I'm good at nothing. Whenever I get into trouble, it seems that Dov is always there watching. Then he and his friends laugh about me. It was such a nice change for him to be nice to me. We had a good time together that evening - after it was all over.

Suddenly, Pokey starts jumping all around and getting excited. As she starts running out of the fort, I hear Michael walking up the front steps. I guess Pokey heard him way before I did. They do say that dogs have great hearing.

Mom lets Michael in. As he enters the front room and starts to say, 'Hello Eli', his eyes get really big. He's looking at my fort creation. "Wow, Eli" he says. "You are one of the most creative people I know. How do you get such fantastic ideas? This fort is awesome."

I'm not sure how to answer Michael. I do get some pretty creative ideas. I don't know how, they just come to me. It's like having a light go 'boing'. Maybe it's because I spend a lot of time putting together these cool 3-D puzzles or building elaborate scenes with my Legos®. It's more fun to put together my own cities and creations than to read or follow the instructions. I imagine that these kinds of activities help me get

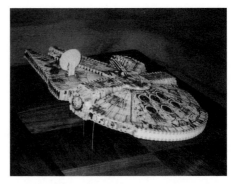

3-D Puzzle of Star Wars Ship, Millennium Falcon

good ideas for creating other things. Besides, I like to build stuff. It's so fun to do things with my hands and to be able to see the neat inventions that appear.

We hang out and have a good time in the fort. After a while, Mom comes in and peeks into our fort, saying, "Hello, Eli. Hello, Michael. This is sure a cool fort you guys have."

"Yeh, it is, isn't it? Eli built it before I got here," says Michael.

Mom tells us it's time to get ready to go to piano. We sadly take down the cool fort, put away the stuff and get into the car.

During the drive, I think about how excited I was as I first started piano. I really felt I could do it. And I did — in the beginning. I really liked all the rhythm activities and I can play a bunch of songs. They sound pretty good. It got hard though when I had to use two hands together.

Michael started at the same time, and now he's so much better than I am. He now plays songs that are much harder than mine are. I didn't realize that I was struggling until I found out how much easier it is for everybody else in the class.

Once again, I feel like here is another thing everyone else is better at. Mom and Dad won't let me quit: they say it's good to stick with it. Hummm, maybe if I promise them I'll take up guitar, they'll let me stop piano lessons. I'll have to think about that.

Prequel: Disappearing Report

Today I come home from school with the babysitter, Maria. She's cool, and I like her. It's fun when this sitter gets me, because we have a snack and I play until she rings a bell. The bell means it's time for me to start homework. Ugh. I have so much more homework now that I'm in fourth grade.

I decide to build a fort in the living room; it's an awesome wonderful fort. Pokey and Peanut come in with me and we have great adventures. We scare away all the enemies: we're the heroes! Just like Georgie, my pet turtle, escapes by pulling his head in his shell, I escape by going into my fort. Inside, I organize my world the way I want. I can be *okay* and I can be like my friends. In my fort, I'm not different from everybody else. I know if I ever leave, I'll have to do my homework. I don't like homework, especially tonight.

I hear the bell ring and ignore it, refusing to come out. Peanut reminds me I really should pay attention to Maria, otherwise Mom will get mad at her. Then Mom probably won't even pay her. I don't want that. I like Maria. So, I find my way out of my wonderful fort.

Once again, my homework is writing. It's always writing. I have to do a one-page report on the state of California. I know all about California. I live here and we've been studying it all week. It's just that I hate writing. Writing is hard. I mix up letters. Spelling is horrible and doesn't seem to make any sense to me. Even when I know all the information, I mix up the facts, especially when I have to write them down.

I don't like being different. I don't like having to work so hard. I work harder than all my friends and my grades aren't nearly as good. Mom says it's because I have a learning disability —this means I learn differently. The official name is *dyslexia,* and many famous and successful people have

Eli

---

dyslexia. My favorite is Robin Williams, because he is left-handed like me. Also, he gets to be in a bunch of really funny movies. He's a lucky guy.

Just because Robin Williams has this thing called *dyslexia* like I do, that doesn't make me feel any better. It especially doesn't make me feel any better when I work so much harder than my friends, but get grades that are worse. My brain is like Swiss cheese: things just fall right out.

As Peanut says, I have to do this report. So, I slowly saunter over to the computer.

Man, this is hard. I know what I want to say, but the words just don't come out. And, then, they don't go on the paper in the right way. I

> Checklist for writing - to give me POWER !!!
>
> 1. Plan
>   a. Plan what I want to say
>   b. Create a mind map
> 2. Organize
>   a. Organize my ideas
>   b. Put them in order and number them
> 3. Write
>   a. Write a topic sentence to introduce
>   b. Write each idea
>   c. Write a conclusion – the summary
> 4. Edit
>   a. Check it over
>   b. Make corrections
> 5. Revise
>   a. Rewrite the final
>   b. Make it neat

just sit there. Then I remember I still have to try and I still have to use my strategies. Where is that checklist Tammy gave me to use?

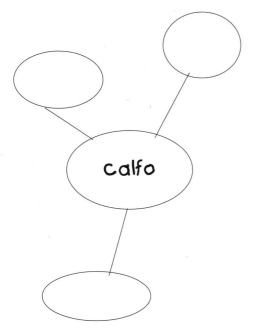

Finally, I find it. I draw a circle in the middle of a page and write 'calfo' in the circle. Then, I think about three main things about California. I draw three more circles and write my three ideas, one in each circle. Now, I am organized. I begin to type. I name and save my report, 'calfor'.

First, I have to type an introduction. Since I like dinosaurs, Tammy explained I should think about a Brachio-

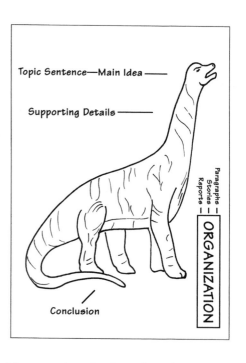

saurus when I write a report. The head is like the introduction which gets my report started. Then, I type a paragraph about each of my ideas in those three smaller circles. These paragraphs are like the long neck of the Brachiosaurus. Its neck holds together its head and connects it all the way to its tail. Tammy says my paragraphs hold together my beginning, the introduction, and my end, the conclusion.

I start to type. Finally, after what seems like a long time, I have a page of stuff about California.

Wow! Can this really be true? Yes, I believe I'm actually

finished. Amazing – it does help to think about each small chunk of the report one at a time -- instead of just thinking about it all. Tammy always says, 'One step at a time'. And, look, it's still light outside. This is indeed miraculous.

Uh-oh – I think that I pushed the wrong button on the computer. Where did everything go? This can't really be happening — it can't be that my report just disappeared into thin air! "UGH!" I scream and run into my fort. It's safe there. Maria calls me but too bad, I'm not coming out.

Eventually, Mom and Dad come home. I hear Maria telling them what happened. She says that she left the computer exactly as it was. Dad sits down at the computer for a bit and then calls, "Hello, hello Eli. Come on out here please."

I slowly edge out of my fort. Dad asks in his soft voice, "Eli, did you save your file when you started your report?" I say, "Yes, but I didn't save anything after the beginning." I feel so awful I just hang my head down. I'm not crying but tears kinda leak out.

Dad says calmly, "Eli, please sit here in this computer chair. Go to your documents' file. Look for your report. Is it there?"

"Wow" I scream. "It's there! Oh Dad, you're magic."

I open the file called "calfor," and, to my surprise, everything is there except the conclusion. This is so amazing. I can't imagine how it happened. Then Dad reminds me about "autosave." I remember now that's why I have to name my file and save it as soon as I start to work.

The conclusion is missing. No sweat. Conclusions are easy; I always do them the same way. I type,

I'd like to visit California. It has many mountains and forests.

Chapter 1: Homework

Homework is definitely the worst part of the day. It takes so long.

All I want to do is finish and play on my computer. I love my computer. I'm a champ at the games where I can either design and control my own city, or games where I can build and create things by solving puzzles. But my parents say I can't play computer until I finish all my homework. And they even check up on me. Bummer.

I wiggle around as I think about my three assignments. I always have more work than other kids in my class. Besides, my daily papers are almost never "good enough" for Teacher. She usually makes me redo them. Not fair.

I worry a lot about going to junior high next year. They're

going to load so much written work on me. There is one good thing about junior high: maybe Sam won't be there. He's the kid in class who teases me the most.

I shake myself to stop dreaming and try to remember what Mom says. Oh yeah, "You don't have to worry about it today. Junior high will come soon enough." I know I need to get to my homework. Every day it's the same dilemma; Should I do the easiest or the hardest assignment first ?

I think I'll start with the one I hate the most. Besides, that's what Mom always says. She even gave me a sign, right here on my wall.

Eli: do the hardest 1st!

Writing is definitely the worst task of all. It's just way too hard to remember all the things I need, like periods and capital letters. Then, it's almost impossible to think about how to spell words when I'm busy trying to think about the story. It's so hard to remember what I'm writing about. I remember a picture I saw in a book about a kid juggling all these balls. The author* explained that juggling is like writing – you have to think about a bunch of pieces all at once.

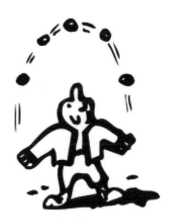

I figure it's easier to write just a few sentences. That doesn't hurt my hand so much either. My teachers complain, but I just keep writing very short stories. After all, teachers don't understand what it's like to struggle and struggle to write and still have the paper turn out sloppy and full of mistakes. They always tell me how messy my papers are. They just can't understand how hard I try. No matter how carefully I work, the words don't look the way they look for the other kids. Sometimes I know how I want the word to look, but it just doesn't turn out that way.

*Based on Mel Levine's discussion in *Keeping A Head in School*

Eli

It's awful to get a paper back with all those red marks. It seems that the teacher wants to make the paper bleed, it's so red. I'm determined when I grow up, I'll never use a red pen!

I remember how much I loved it when my second grade class read stories from *Old Mother West Wind**. Those animals had so many adventures and the stories were so whimsical. I can think about them for hours and create great adventures with those amazing characters. I like them so much that I even wrote my own story about Old Mother West Wind and some chicks.

I lean back in my chair and think about how really good I feel about the stories I wrote way back in second grade. They were longer than the stories I create now for class. I was actually interested in constructing stories back then. It was fun to do all that imagining.

Old Mother West Wind, by Thorton Burgess.

I have a few favorite stories, but I know I can never share them. Teachers will just complain about spelling, capital letters, and punctuation marks, and they'll mark up my story with that horrible red pen. I always have two secret stories in my pocket. One is about the chicks and Old Mother West Wind, and the other is about a haunted house.

I reach into my pocket for the stories*. Maybe one of them will give me an idea for the story I have to write for class tomorrow. I sure hate to write. I pull the ragged, dog-eared papers from my pocket. They are so beat up that pretty soon I won't be able to read either one. Maybe I can sneak to a copy machine some day.

Reading about the animals in my Old Mother West Wind story gives me an idea.

I decide I'll write about being a dog or a dolphin. I'll call my story, "Life of a Eli."

*Eli's two favorite stories are in Appendix 1.

Eli

Life of a Eli

I hate my school life because it is unfar and no fun being how I am.I cam not right ore spell ore math ore stody. And eseshaly the warst is that I get hert all the time and In not good at any spart.I amly have three friends but they might be ysing me to amd hate me.I cant do emy thinyng weth out losine a freind ore herting my self.I d rather be a dog ar a dalfen.I d be loved more and have more frend.I d be happy.

(Translation: I hate my school life because it is unfair and no fun being how I am. I cannot write or spell or [do] math or study. And especially the worst is that I get hurt all the time and I'm not good at any sport. I only have three friends but they might be using me too and hate me. I can't do anything without losing a friend or hurting myself. I'd rather be a dog or a dolphin. I'd be loved more and have more friends. I'd be happy.)

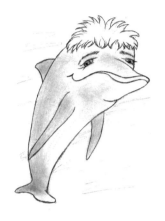

Now that's done. The worst part is finally over. I'm so relieved. I think about how much fun I'd have being a dolphin swimming in a deep blue sea. Or, jumping up high, trying to reach the bright yellow sun. I'm so fast and I discover so many glorious things. There's this great big group of fish. What's a big group called? Oh yeah, it's a school of fish. Whoops, thinking of a school of fish reminds me of school - and homework.

Time to return to my yucky homework. I rework the class math problems that were done wrong. That actually doesn't take too long and is fairly easy. Cool. That's done.

Next I have to create sentences for my spelling words. I saunter over to use Mom's computer, stopping to say hi to each of my animals. The computer's cool because it puts a

Eli

funny line under words I spell wrong. For some papers, when it's real important, I look up misspelled words on my electronic speller. I'm glad Teacher is okay with me typing my spelling sentences - it's so much easier for my fingers, because they cramp up when I use a pencil for too long.

My electronic speller is a Franklin Speller®, and it lets me punch in the word the way it sounds. Then it lists words that match. I never know which word to choose but when I push the "say" button, the Franklin reads me the choices. Upon hearing each word, I can choose the right one. Since I have to use something, the Franklin's a good option. I like it because its robotic voice is so funny. Sometimes I just play with it to hear that funny sound.

I start to type my sentences. My first word is 'vibrant'. That word reminds me of one of my posters. So I write,

The dulfin jumps in the viberant blu sky.

I also have a cool shark poster that shows bunches of sharks bearing their rows of long pointed teeth. This poster is next to my jungle poster that has so many bright colorful birds. They're flying all over and some are off in the distance. Those look like squiggly lines, like on my computer. Oops, distracted again - back to my sentences.

Wildlife is awesome! My walls are so covered with animal posters that many of them are tacked up on the ceiling. That's handy, because anytime I look up I can just immerse myself into my wonderful animal posters.

I'm lucky to also have live animals in my room to keep me company. I wonder if all parents are so understanding. Mom always says it's okay for me to have pets as long as I remember to be responsible with them.

My three family dogs are usually curled up under my table. In a five-gallon fish tank live my four newts. They're

Eli

unusual enough that many of my friends have never seen one before. My sand crabs hide out in a 10-gallon tank. It's fun to take them out and watch them play. When they walk on the tile floor their feet go "clip, click, clack."

Georgie, my pet box turtle, has a tank all to himself. I enjoy playing with him outside. It's so neat how Georgie can 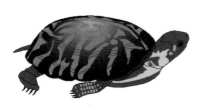 pull his head and feet into his shell and escape from the outside world. I like Georgie a lot, and I often wonder what it would be like to escape like that.

Then there are my hamsters, They're my favorite pets. I started out with three hamsters, two females and a male. Now there are babies all over the place. Every so often, I gather up the oldest babies and take them to a pet store. The store gives me credit to buy food and more tunnels, wheels, and curvy passages for my Habitrails®. That's the best kind of hamster cage because I can rearrange the trails and tunnels so many different ways. I'm proud of my huge Habitrails®. They go all over my room, even over and under the precious treasures on my big table. My hamsters sure are lucky to have all those tunnels and secret passageways.

Passageways are neat. I often wonder what kind of passage is in the forest behind my house. I'm glad my family just moved to this neat neighborhood. Other people live all around me, but not behind me. That's where the forest is. It's a mysterious forest that spreads out as far as I can see.

I look out the window at the forest and dream about exploring it. "Maybe there are secret passages there." I hope I get a chance to explore it soon.

Oh, oh. Mom's calling, "Eli, how are you doing?" Well, back to those spelling sentences.

Chapter 2: The Meeting

It's Wednesday morning. In my classroom, I look up at the ceiling, daydreaming about the coming holiday weekend. I'm so glad it's some president's birthday or something like that. There's no school on Friday. I can't wait to be free. I only have to get through today and tomorrow, and then I can have a big three-day weekend with no writing to do.

When it's my turn, I shuffle to Teacher's desk and hand her my story. I wiggle from one foot to the other while she reads it. She starts talking to me. Uh-oh - here comes.

"Eli", she says, "this story isn't good enough. Your paper is way too messy. You must have rushed again. I always tell you to slow down. I want you to write it over. If you need more time, you can use your recess time."

I slowly stumble back to my desk to rewrite my dolphin story. Rewriting my homework makes me feel sad and stupid.

I try to recopy my story very carefully. At least I don't have to worry about what I have to say. With one minute to spare before recess, I carry the finished creation back to Teacher. Oh no! What's that? She doesn't even try to read it. She just glances at the paper and says, "Eli, you need to write it again. This one is the sloppiest of all. Didn't you even try?" She doesn't believe how hard I worked. That's as bad as when kids in my class tease me.

I'm so crushed it's hard to breathe. Oh gee. I can feel my eyes stinging. I gulp. Before I know it, I burst into tears. This is probably the most embarrassing thing that can happen. I turn to run out of the room. I just want to keep going even though I don't know where. The tears keep flowing as I race out the door, feeling more and more frustrated. Soon I'm sobbing so hard I can hardly see. Running down the hallway, I crash smack into Principal.

Principal starts to holler, "No running!" but then she looks at me and must have realized how upset I am. She sends me to her office and goes to talk to Teacher.

"Uh-oh! Now I'm really in trouble!" I think as I cringe, still sobbing.

Principal calls Mom. I can hear a little through the door. She's asking Mom to come to school. Oh great! Another conference. There have already been so many conferences. I know they don't do any good. No one ever listens. I'm scared. What's going to happen now?

Soon Mom arrives. We all meet in an empty classroom: Teacher, Principal, Mom, and even me. I wonder who's teaching our class. Walking in, I'm thinking this is probably a waste of time. Why did they even bother to include me?

Teacher first says, "I know how hard writing is for you, Eli, and I'm sorry I was insensitive. It's no excuse, but I was having a rough day and was distracted. I didn't mean to upset you."

Oh my. Am I hearing correctly?

Then Mom talks. She doesn't need to hear why I started crying and running. She already knows how hard I work and how frustrating it all is. With everyone listening, she explains that I'm not lazy or defiant (that means I'm not trying to be bad). I have something weird called *dysgraphia*.

Eli

Dysgraphia means that a person doesn't mean to be sloppy, but it's hard for the hands to cooperate with the brain when trying to write. The more that is written, the more tired one's hand gets. The more tired a hand gets, the sloppier the writing. Mom shows them a book and a bunch of papers that tell all about this mystery called *dysgraphia*. Mom says it's related to my dyslexia. This seems to help everyone understand better. Principal and Teacher take a lot of notes.

I have to admit, Teacher is a nice lady. I remember that we do have fun in class and we often create awesome projects. I like the projects.

Then Teacher asks me some questions, like how long it took me to write the dolphin story and how I came up with the idea. She is actually listening to my explanations. Wow. Then she promises to stop bugging me so much about neatness if I agree always to try my best. Also, I can now use a computer whenever there's a whole lot of writing to do. I promise to try my best and promise not to run out of class again.

We then set up the 'red card plan'. With this plan, I get to keep a red card at my desk. Whenever I feel very, very frustrated and want to escape, I give the teacher the special card and then go to Principal's office.

This plan makes me feel like they're trying to understand me. I don't even need to say anything before leaving the room. Principal's office will be my timeout place until I can work again.

This red card plan is great. I like the idea of having an escape place where I can regain control. Besides, it will help Teacher remember that I really am trying my best.

I still wish that I could write like some of the other kids.

Eli

And I wish I didn't have *dysgraphia*. I especially wish that I wasn't different. For the first time in a long, long time, I feel hopeful about school again, at least a little bit. I'm still scared. Will my friends continue to tease me?

Chapter 3: The Cave

Finally, it's Friday. The big day is here at last!

Michael, my best friend, is coming over. We always have a grand time together. The doorbell rings and Michael is here. Oh no. I can't believe my eyes. Sam is here, too.

I don't like Sam, because he always teases me. He calls me names like, "the sloppy one" and "lazy" and, worst of all, "slow poke." Because of Sam, I often rush through my class work, and this makes my writing sloppier than ever. It's so important not to be the last one done. It's more important to finish before Sam, even if the work is wrong and will need to be redone at home later.

And now, here is Sam at my front door with my best friend, Michael. I groan and don't know what to do.

Eli

Finally, Sam says, "Hey Eli. Let us in." I step aside and Michael and Sam enter. I don't understand why Sam is here. I guess it'll be okay, as long as he doesn't see my bedroom. I don't want him to tell everyone at school that my awesome room is 'stupid' or something like that.

Michael says, "Hi, there. Sam's mom had to go away, so Sam came over and here we are."

We hang out in the yard for a while, but that soon gets boring. When Sam suggests we explore the forest, I hesitate. Mom says I'm not supposed to go there. I definitely don't want to give Sam a reason to call me 'chicken'. I say, 'okay,' because I am curious about what's beyond those first trees. So, how can I resist?

We walk into the forest. The trees are huge. The forest is so thick that the sun can't get through to the ground. This makes it pretty dark. We realize we need a light, so I run back and grab a flashlight from Dad's toolbox.

The three of us then enter the woods.

We carefully pick our way through the trees. Some heavy branches hang low and leaves brush our faces as we move along. Roots catch our toes and cause us to stumble. Finally, we see an opening right in front of us. Can it be a cave?

Michael and I don't want to go in. But Sam is acting so tough and sure of himself that I don't dare suggest going home. I consider making the offer to stand guard outside the entrance, but Sam is already

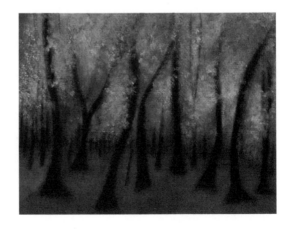

Eli

slipping into the cave. The way Sam disappears so quickly reminds me of Georgie pulling into his shell. I think, "Hmmm, this cave might be a good hideout and a fun secret place." I guess I'll go in too.

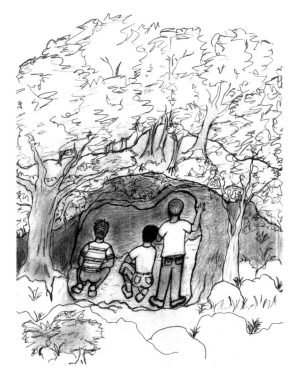

It's darker and scarier in the cave than in the forest. We're glad to have a flashlight. There are so many turns and twisting paths. Some places are really low, forcing us to crawl. Strange sounds are all around, and it is hard to tell what the sounds are or even where they're coming from. In just a few minutes, the exciting adventure begins to seem like a 'not-so-hot' idea. Michael whispers to me, "Hey, do you think we'll be able to find our way out of here?"

After a while, the ceiling of the cave becomes so high we can hardly see it. We sit down to rest and Sam suggests we tell scary stories. Michael suggests we head back. I am so relieved Michael said that. I want to go back, too.

As I get up and start walking back, Sam groans and says, "You guys are wimps."

Suddenly, a small furry bat darts through the beam of our flashlight. Sam yelps and bumps into me, causing the flashlight to fall and turn off. It's suddenly darker than the darkest night. As Michael and I search for the flashlight, we hear a soft whimpering sound and start to get scared.

I'm relieved when I finally find the flashlight. I turn it on.

Eli

As I look around, I realize there is nothing to fear. The sound is from Sam. He's curled up on the floor of the cave crying. Michael and I try to tell him it's just an old bat and nothing to be afraid of. Sam doesn't seem to hear us.

Michael and I know we have to get Sam out of the cave. We start to go out, dragging him with us. In all the confusion, we can't find the path to lead us out. We try one and then another. We keep hitting dead ends or we end up back in the same place. Michael suggests we rest. Sam collapses.

Then I remember my gnome. I haven't thought about him for a long, long time.

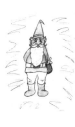 Way back in kindergarten, things got tough at school because pictures and letters were hard to make and ended up so messy. I didn't feel too good about myself, and I imagined a small gnome friend to help me stay calm. He always made me feel

better because he reminded me that I could do lots of things really well. I call him 'Peanut' because he is so small.

I close my eyes for a moment and wish hard. Sure enough, Peanut appears on my shoulder. No one else can see him. No one else can hear him. Peanut is my secret.

I listen as Peanut whispers in my ear, "Remember helping your mom find the car in the mall parking lot? You always know where she parks the car. Remember your dad telling about the time you showed your grandpa the road to your mom's work? You were only three. You're good at finding your way, and you can find your way out of this cave."

I turn to Sam and Michael and tell them, "Come on! I can get us out of here." Sam doesn't stop crying but he seems to calm down a little bit. He scrambles to his feet and willingly walks with me and Michael.

Eli

Peanut points to a rock. "Remember that stone there?" he asks me. "You thought it looks like a dolphin." And I remember. We turn down the path that goes right by the dolphin rock.

A little further, Peanut points to another rock. "Remember that one over there that looks like a monkey?" he asks. I remember.

"This way!" I tell the others as they start to turn down a different pathway.

"Hey," says Sam, "how do you know which way to go?"

I'm not sure what to say. With my terrific imagination, I can make up wonderful stories; but I don't ever share them with other kids. They might think I'm a dork or something.

Something has changed. I have seen Sam cry. Sam is a real person, not just a mean bully. He can get scared, just like anyone else. Maybe it is safe for me to share my secret. Michael has never made fun of me before, so I know I can trust him now.

I decide to take a chance and tell them about Peanut, even though I've never told anyone before. It's so scary, but I do it anyway.

I tell Sam and Michael about how Peanut helped me in kindergarten. "I forgot about him for a while. Maybe I was too upset about school to remember, or maybe I thought I was too old to think about gnomes. I don't know. But I remembered him today. And I know we can make it out of here."

The three of us now arrive at a spot where two dark tunnels come together. Peanut reminds me about the shark-shaped root growing on the right near the top of the tunnel. We look at that root and move on in that direction.

Eli

"Tell us more about your gnome," says Michael.

"Yeah, there are lots of times I could use a gnome," Sam adds.

I'm surprised. I never dreamed that other kids might need to be reminded of stuff they are good at to help them when they struggle. I begin to describe Peanut in detail.

"He's a small guy, about the size of a peanut, two or three inches high. He can be any size he wants. He lives with his tribe and he comes to help me whenever I need him. He's the one who helps switch on the light in my head. You know the imaginary light I mean, the ideas that just pop into your head. I think they're like a light bulb. When I'm frustrated, sometimes my ideas just get blocked. Then Peanut reminds me about all the stuff I can do. You know how your parents always say they're proud of you and you have lots of talent. Sometimes I think they're just trying to make me feel good. Peanut reminds me what I'm good at and that helps.

"I wish you could see him. He has a big white moustache that sticks out at the sides and a long white beard that hangs down over his belly. His fat belt has a toolkit so he can help me fix all kinds of things. You know how I'm real good at fixing stuff. He wears a big, tall pointed blue hat and his bushy hair sticks out from underneath it."

"Wow, wouldn't it be cool if everyone could have a gnome like that to talk to?" Michael grins. "I want one!"

Sam agrees that having a gnome can be useful. "I think my gnome will be a little younger and dress better." We all laugh. We aren't nearly as scared.

As we walk and talk, I continue to notice things we

Eli

passed when we entered the cave. It doesn't take long to retrace our steps to the rock shaped like a turtle near the mouth of the cave.

"Hey! Light!" shouts Michael. "We made it!"

We run all the way back through the rest of the forest to my house. Sam, who's in the lead, stops suddenly when he catches sight of my mom standing in the yard looking our way.

"Uh-oh, Eli, is your mom gonna be mad?" he asks fearfully.

"Looks like it. I'm not supposed to go in the forest. She'll go easy on you guys; you're guests," I say, hoping I'm right. Maybe she will cut them some slack; they aren't her kids.

We receive the expected lecture but nothing seems as bad after being so scared in the cave. We also have to clear off the patio and clean up the yard while Mom fixes lunch.

Chapter 4: The Cando Tribe

During lunch, I tell Mom about all that happened in the cave, only leaving out the part about Sam crying. I even tell her Peanut showed up again. When Sam and Michael tell their ideas about wanting a gnome, she looks thoughtful. After we finish eating, she says,

"Peanut comes from the Cando Gnome Tribe. His real name is Eli Youcan. I've got a feeling that you boys each have your own gnome. Michael, I'll bet if you try, you'll find a Michael Youcan waiting to help you and remind you of things you can do well. And Sam, your Sam Youcan can be dressed differently and be more modern, but he's there, waiting for you to find him. What he looks like doesn't matter.

"You know, boys, we all have a little voice in our heads.

Eli

Do you ever talk to yourself, like when you're doing a math problem or figuring something out? That little voice is like Eli Youcan's voice."

Sam and Michael are quiet. Then they say they're not too sure how to go about finding their own gnomes. So, Mom offers to help.

She starts by asking Michael what he can do really well. He thinks for a while and then says, "I know. I'm a good speller. I almost always get A's on my spelling tests."

"Good!" Mom says. "What else can you do?"

"That's all," says Michael. "Math and reading are hard and I'm not too good at sports."

"What's your best subject in school after spelling?" Mom prompts.

"Well . . . oh, wait. I got an A in science. I guess I'm pretty good at that."

"Keep going," Mom encourages.

"I'm good at understanding what I read. I don't read too fast, but I remember the ideas. And I've got more merit badges than all the other kids in my Scout troop."

"Excellent, Michael. That's exactly what I mean." Mom turns to Sam. "Okay, Sam, what about you?"

Sam has already figured it out. "Well, I don't get history and I don't build stuff. I write okay and I pitch for my baseball team," he volunteers.

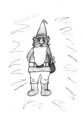

"And?" coaxes Mom.

"I'm great at drawing, and I can ride my skateboard better than most of my friends," he boasts.

Eli

"You all have many things to be proud of, boys," Mom tells us. "Do you ever think about these things when you try to do something really hard, or when you're struggling doing something new?"

"No," Michael and Sam admit.

"Well, that's when you need to remember more than ever what you're good at. Everyone has some things we do really well and other things we don't find easy. And that's okay. We're all different and have different talents and skills. If everyone was the same as everyone else, life could be pretty dull."

We all agree.

Mom tells us about famous people who had problems with different subjects in school, but who also had talents that were really special. Some entertainers are Tom Cruise,

Tommie Smothers, and Robin Williams. Scientists include Alexander Graham Bell, Thomas Edison, and Albert Einstein. And there are others like the writer, Hans Christian Anderson, and the artist, Pablo Picasso.

She adds, "The important thing is that they work with the skills and talents that they have, and they don't think they are dumb just because some tasks are tough.

"This is how Eli's gnome helps him. Eli is good at finding his way around places. It was Eli who got you out of the cave today. The gnome is really a part of Eli. It's his inside voice that reminds him of all the talents he has that make him who he is. Do you see? It's not how you turn on that little light in your head, but it is important to remember it when you need reminding that you really are a great person!"

Sam and Michael have nearly an hour before leaving. I feel safe now in asking Sam if he wants to see my room.

Eli

"Yeah, he's got the greatest room!" says Michael.

"Okay," Sam says. We head down the hall.

When Sam sees my amazing pad, he doesn't laugh or tease me. "Whoa! This is really wild," he exclaims. He checks out all the animals and the twists and turns of the Habitrails®. He thinks they're cool. But what really catches his eye is the line of huge 3-D puzzles on a shelf along one wall.

"Hey, did you build these all by yourself?" he asks me.

"Yeah. They took a long time, but they were fun," I answer. "It's weird that Mom and Dad

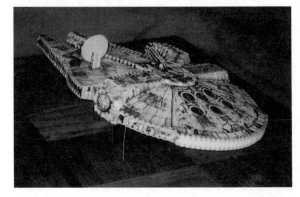

can't help me with stuff like this. They even have trouble with plain old flat puzzles on the table!"

"Man, me, too. I struggle to put together regular puzzles when the pieces are this small," Sam says. "These are great. I like the Star Wars Ship the best."

"Thanks," I grin. Sam is turning out to be an okay guy after all. I don't think Sam will pick on me at school after our adventure. Well, I hope.

We all learned different things today, probably more than we would have at school. We discovered a lot about each other, and even more important, we discovered a great deal about ourselves!

And, the Cando Gnome Tribe adds two new members to its group.

Chapter 5: School

Monday soon comes and it's time for school again. I'm worried, thinking, "What if Sam forgets he was nice to me and starts teasing me again?" When I see Sam at school, he comes over with a big smile to "hi". My fears are relieved, at least for a while.

The bell rings, and we all go into class. The first assignment is to write about our weekend.

"Oh no!" I think, "Here we go again!"

Sam leans over and to my surprise whispers, "Eli, I know you hate writing, but remember you have strengths too." Then I smile, take a deep breath, and think about my strategies. If I just take one step at a time, maybe I can manage this.

I write my ideas down:

✔ Sam and Mikel cam ovre

✔ we wen into the fouris behind my hous

✔ we fond a cav

✔ we went in

✔ we explored

I decide to leave out the part about getting lost, Sam getting scared, and about Peanut helping us. That's personal stuff.

I write about the five ideas I listed. It is rather short, but it does tell about my weekend. After I'm done, I go back over the story and add some capital letters and periods. Then I try and find words that may be spelled wrong. I put a line under these words, and maybe I will look them up later on my

Eli

Franklin. There are so many underlines.

When I hand my paper to Teacher, I explain that the underlines are words I'm not sure about. I don't want her to have a chance to say I didn't try. Instead, she smiles and says, "Thank you, Eli. I can see that you worked hard on this." Wow! No complaints. This is amazing and unbelievable.

I sometimes wish things could be perfect for me and my friends. But life is never perfect. I think about the red card plan I can use whenever I get too frustrated. As it turns out, I never even use it. Just knowing that I can use it is enough.

Michael, Sam, and I all began to notice a difference in school this year. A complex math problem doesn't seem so overwhelming if we remind ourselves of something else we like to do or are good at, and especially if we think about the problem one step at a time. When we feel calm instead of frustrated, it is actually easier to get through the work.

By the end of the school year, I realize that Michael still reads slower than some other kids and he will never be a star football player in the NFL. He's just too slow and clumsy. But he can spell and he always understands what he reads. Sam probably won't ever build houses or write a history book. But he draws all kinds of wonderful pictures for the class bulletin board.

And me? Well, I probably won't write any kind of book. I still don't like to write, but I feel that at least my teacher understands—a little. Besides, boy, can I fix things, and I sure can find my way around.

Throughout the year, I notice other kids in my class who also have a hard time in some subjects but are good at other things. Maybe I'm not so different after all. I realize that everyone is different in his or her own way. I finally understand what it means when people tell me, "we have all kinds of minds." We're not all the same.

I begin to agree. Yep, it is good to have all kinds of minds— because we really are all different. It keeps life interesting.*

Who knows? Maybe someday I will fix computers for people who do like to write. Maybe someday I will even have a computer that will let me talk while it does all the typing.

*Refer to, *All Kinds of Minds* by Mel Levine

Epilogue

It's hard to believe I've already made it through 2 1/2 years of college. Here I am with the same struggles I had way back in elementary school; what can I write about? It is always so hard to get my ideas. Then comes the struggle to organize those ideas. It never gets easier.

I'm majoring in computers but I still have to get through all these required courses like math and English. Technology advances allow me to use voice-activated software to talk into a headset while the computer program types what I say. I like my Dragon Naturally Speaking® program. Even so, I still need to be careful about spelling and editing my papers, or have someone else go over them. I still think about the old Brachiosaurus that Tammy taught me way back when. I know that writing will never be easy; it will take me more time, more effort, and more work than it will my peers.

Eli

Our English class has been working on allegories, which I have been assigned to write. An allegory is an expression or story that uses symbolic fictional figures and draws generalizations about human existence. It can be about any subject, but has to use animals or imaginary characters.

I think about that time in 6th grade when I got into a fight with a kid during recess. We were playing basketball and this kid kept pushing everybody. Finally, I pushed him back, resulting in a fight between us. A teacher broke it up. It was embarrassing when tears fell from my eyes even though I told them I wasn't crying.

As a result, Teacher and Principal told me I had to sit on the bench during recess for a whole week or take another option. At that point, because I was quite bored of sitting on that slab of wood, I decided to take the other option. They asked me to tutor a kindergarten kid during recess. I didn't know if I could do it, but anything was better than sitting on the bench.

I soon found out that I enjoyed working with the kindergarten kid because being able to help someone else made me feel smart. Besides, that kid said I was really helping him a lot. Imagine!

I wish I could get out of having to write this allegory. Like that time in class when Teacher announced we would now all read our weekly state reports aloud in class, right after the whole school assembly on our state. That day, at the end of the assembly, I noticed that the assembly teacher was having a hard time closing up the projector. I couldn't understand why she was having so much trouble. It's really quite easy. I hung back and offered to help her.

I could easily figure out most things mechanical, even way back then. So, from then on, it became my job to work on the projector for the assembly and I merely handed in my state report to Teacher. They also allowed me to help set up and put away the chairs, which kept me out of class even

Eli

more. I liked it and knew I was being helpful. I felt valued and useful. Most importantly, the other kids didn't have to listen to me read my report aloud in class.

I know my thinking is different from other people. So many times, having a different thinking pattern gets me in trouble and it definitely causes me to have to work harder. Other times, being different is like having a gift.

Working with machines is one of my gifts and Mom always says I'm real intuitive with machines. Back then, I wasn't sure what 'intuitive' meant. Now I understand that it means I can figure out almost any machine and rarely read the instructions. I used to think Mom and Dad were just not very smart about machines. Then, when I saw that many of the teachers also struggled to set up machines, especially projectors and computers, I began to realize that some adults do actually have trouble trying to understand such devices; they don't see them the same way I do. Maybe that's what intuitive about machines means: machines just make sense to me, even computers.

When our sixth grade class first got computers, I was the one chosen to set them up. Then in seventh grade, the librarian asked me to come in and set up the new computer lab when they changed all their computers. I then become the library aide.

Sometimes people acknowledge my gifts and talents. When that happens I get conflicting feelings. On one hand, it feels rather good to receive acknowledgment. On the other hand, I always wonder if they're just trying to make me feel better. There's a nagging question in my head: Am I really just lazy and using this 'learning difference' as an excuse? Sometimes I feel so insecure. So many people, my teachers, my psychologist, and my parents, tell me I'm not lazy and that I just learn differently. My major worry is a nagging doubt if this is true, or if maybe I am just stupid or lazy.

Eli

Sometimes I feel guilty when I receive special privileges, questioning if I really deserve them. I know I am a 'jack of all trades'. I can usually pick up and do anything pretty well. Maybe I'm just being lucky and in the right spot when something needs to be done.

At my elementary school graduation, it was tradition for the faculty to present an award to the one graduating student who made the most progress and worked hardest in making that progress. I never expected to be the one chosen at my graduation. I was shocked upon hearing my name called.

I recall how confusion set in as I realized that the whole school was clapping for me. It was a wonderful feeling that people were actually acknowledging that I tried hard. On the other hand, I was so unsure as to whether I deserved it.

In spite of my learning struggles, I made good grades throughout middle school and even in high school.

My parents and I learned the importance of sharing information about my learning difference with each one of my
teachers. Through communication, most teachers appreciate
how hard I need to work. This is important, especially in
college.

If I could get through all those years of school, surely I
can write one more paper, like this allegory.

Thinking, thinking. I think of an eagle.

Finally, I write the story, *When the Eagles Could Not
Fly**. Now, I'll have something to turn in tomorrow.

A few years later, while sitting listening to speeches at
my college graduation, I think again about that allegory I
wrote about the eagles. It was a good way to explain the

*Eli's story, *When the Eagles Could Not Fly* follows

need to accept others as they are, as well as the need to value each person's strengths. I guess it's considered a completed allegory, but I never developed the ending the way I originally had in mind.

I remember my brain was getting exhausted pulling together everything I needed to pull together to create the story. So, when I reached a point that I felt I couldn't go on any more, I just found a way to sum up the story. My intention had been to expand more at the end, using greater description to explain how society went bad. I would have liked more depth describing the situation the world would be in when the island society becomes devoid of all kinds of minds. That sure would be a big mess.

It is my hope that teachers, parents and other students will realize that everyone has his or her own set of strengths and weaknesses. It is indeed true that we have all kinds of minds and all kinds of talents.

When The Eagles Could Not Fly*

The Turtles
An old race that could easily be misled and thought of themselves as the wisest
Skills: Good problem solvers, good counters and organizers

The Eagles
A proud race that took pride in everything they did, and did not talk much
Skills: Good flyers, good vision

The Monkeys
A selfish race that only looked out for themselves
Skills: Good climbers, collectors, and builders

The Ostriches
A shy race that always did whatever they were told
Skills: Fast runners. A good jester

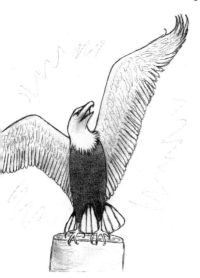

On an island in the middle of the ocean was a great land. On this land lived Turtles, Eagles, Monkeys, and Ostriches. All the animals lived on

*Eli's allegory written in college

the island in peace, each doing their own jobs. The Turtles organized and distributed the food and solved problems. The Eagles flew around the island to watch for enemies. The Monkeys climbed trees to collect food and built houses. And the Ostriches delivered packages and entertained everyone in their own special way. Everything worked out nicely until one day when the Turtles decided that since there had never been any enemies to their island, the Eagles were not contributing much to the community; they felt there must be a change.

The Turtles called all the animals on the island to an important meeting. Once everyone had arrived they explained their new idea about how the Eagles needed a new job since they did not seem to be doing much. All the animals listened intently to the Turtles since they were the oldest and the wisest of the animals. So in the end it was decided that the Eagles would now help out the Monkeys and Ostriches by collecting some of the food and delivering some of the packages. The meeting ended and the Turtles crawled away, the Monkeys swung away, the Ostriches ran away, and the Eagles flew away to start their new job.

The Eagles did not mind their new jobs; in fact they were very good at them—even better—than the Monkeys and Ostriches. Once the Monkeys and Ostriches realized this fact they became scared and decided they must do something about it. They thought that if the Turtles realized the Eagles accomplished their jobs better, that they would become jobless and receive no more food. After many secret meetings between the Monkeys and Ostriches they developed a plan. The Monkeys started sabotaging the food that the Eagles brought to the Turtles; and the Ostriches did the same to the packages delivered by the Eagles (but the Eagles knew nothing of the sabotaging).

After a few weeks the Turtles called another meeting and all the animals came.

"We have been noticing that the Eagles are having problems with their new jobs, The food they bring is rotten and the packages are delivered broken," announced the Turtles.

"YES," cried out the Monkeys. "It is because they are FLYING that the food spoils. They do not know how to protect it and they do not know that it must be carried by foot once picked."

"That is right," the Ostriches spoke out next. "They carelessly fly around not taking care of the packages they deliver and they do not know that they must be carefully delivered by foot."

"We see the problem now, and the solution is simple, unless the Eagles have something to add," the Turtles spoke out. The Eagles were so confused about what was going on. They had thought that their flying ability helped keep the food fresh by getting it to the Turtles quickly, and the packages were kept safe from the pounding of running feet. They could not speak out on their behalf since they did not know what was going on. The Turtles, not hearing a response from the Eagles, relayed their solution.

"Since you have nothing to say about the situation we will solve it. All of the other animals seem to be good at their jobs, and they do not fly. So it seems clear to us that flying is the cause of the problem. So, this skill shall not be practiced on this island from now on. The

Eagles will keep their jobs but must accomplish them without flying. If there is nothing more to say this meeting is ended."

The Eagles were stunned. They could not believe what had just happened. First they found out that they had been doing their jobs poorly, and then they were banned from flying. The Eagles were proud animals, and did not suspect they had been sabotaged. So, they sadly accepted the new rules, since they did not want to be causing the food to go bad or the packages to break. So the meeting ended and the Turtles crawled away. The Monkeys swung away and the Ostriches ran away, both pleased that their plan had worked out. The Eagles slowly walked away to start the new way of doing their jobs.

Three months passed and the Eagles slowly became depressed and seemed to start needing more food from the Turtles. But since they had to do all of the jobs by foot they were very slow, and the Turtles would only give them food after they did a certain amount of work. So they started to become sick. Four months after the new laws started, all of the Eagles were sick and weak and did not do much to help out the

Monkeys or Ostriches. So the Turtles called for another meeting to decide what they were going to do.

"We have two problems to talk about today," the Turtles started out the meeting; "first is the problem with the eagles not doing their part, and second, someone is stealing food." All the Animals started talking at once. They all knew the Eagles had been asking for more food but were denied since they had not helped out very much. Quickly, they all turned the blame on to the Eagles for stealing food.

"It must be the Eagles," shouted the Monkeys and Ostriches. "They were denied more food, so they are stealing it."

"It seems clear to us, too," the Turtles announced. "The Eagles have been a problem for some time now and are now hurting our community and must be banished."

The Eagles were too weak to complain or defend themselves, and so they were all put on a boat and sent off into the ocean as their punishment and banishment.

They floated in the ocean for weeks until one day they floated back to the island by chance and the Turtles instructed the Monkeys and Ostriches to nurse the Eagles back to health. They had little food left because of a rodent infestation that was eating all their food, but they gave all they could to the Eagles. The Eagles soon regained their strength and were told they must start flying.

The Turtles soon realized that before when Eagles were flying on the island they would see rodents and eat them as they did their jobs. This was why they did not need as much food before. Then once they could not fly, they could not find the rodents to eat and so they needed more food. Since the Eagles were not eating the rodents, they started to infest the island and steal the food under the Turtles' noses. This was explained to the Eagles and the Turtles begged their forgiveness. The Monkeys and Ostriches also confessed about how they had sabotaged them before and they too begged their forgiveness.

Eli

The Eagles decided to forgive everyone and were given their original jobs back, since it was now clear that the Eagles had the most important job of protecting the island from enemies, including rodents. The Turtles decided that they would not ever jump to conclusions or try to decide what was better for the other animals. They now understood how important it was that they were all different and all had their own methods for accomplishing their jobs. The community realized that it was okay to do things differently. Even though the Eagles appeared to have an "easy" job, theirs was actually the most important of all.

MORAL:

Accept differences: everyone has their own talents.

Appendix 1

The chicks cracked eggs*

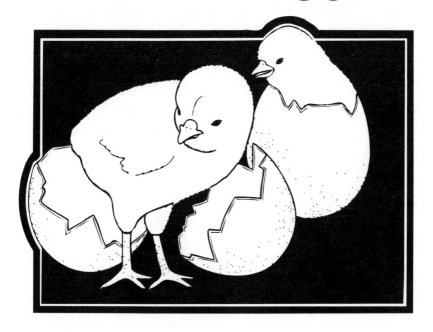

*Written by Eli in the second grade

Eli

Once upon atime a Mrs. Red wing had lade six
gold eggs. It was a suny day. She was very happy
very happy in dead. She was sining a happy song
and wen it was night she exedent brok three
eggs. She only had three left. She was happy and
sad. In the morning the eggs wer jumping and
three yellow chicks came peping theiy wir
hongry. She did not no war to get baby food she
ast Old Mother West Wind she sade It wod be at
the grshry store So she went and bot 100 botels
of baby food wal the babys war eating she nankd
them Eli was the dark yellwe won and Michael was
the lite yellwe won. And Greg wos the metean
eyllwe won. The chicks wor happy with thar
names. Eli and Mickael wir twins theiy owas got
lost and Greg and Mrs. Red Wing hat to lock for
Eli and Mickael. They played with Greg all the
time they had lots of fon togeter. Greg ate a
lot of food he wos fat. Bot Eli and Mickael ha t
ate they war vary sciny you can see right throw
them and you can hadly see them and one day Eli
and Mickael got fat thay ate more ten Greg.

Translation:

Once upon a time, a Mrs. Red Wing had laid six gold eggs. It was a sunny day. She was very happy, very happy indeed. She was singing a happy song and when it was night she accidently broke three eggs. She only had three left. She was happy and sad. In the morning, the eggs were jumping and three yellow chicks came peeping (out). They were hungry. She didn't know where to get baby food. She asked Old Mother West Wind. She said it would be at the grocery store. So she went and bought 100 bottles of baby food. While the babies were eating she named them. Eli was the dark yellow one and Michael was the light yellow one. And Greg was the medium yellow one. The chicks were happy with their names. Eli and Michael were twins. They always got lost and Greg and Mrs. Red Wing had to look for Eli and Michael. They played with Greg all the time. They had lots of fun together. Greg ate a lot of food. He was fat. But Eli and Michael hated to eat. They were very skinny. You can see right through them and you can hardly see them. And one day Eli and Michael got fat. They ate more than Greg.

Appendix 2

The hotid hows*

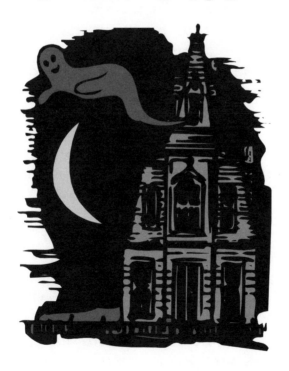

*Written by Eli in the second grade

Eli

Me and Mickael were working down the lon little
path it was raining a omst the mitel of the
night we were comeing home from a party A long
came Jimmy The Skunk He sed thar was a hotid
hows down the rad we went to see the ran wos
beat against the old old howse. The wind howled
through the broken windows. A flash lit up the
rooms. We saw bats. Then we herd thunder and the
sound of foot steps on the stars. We did not
dard to took and som wan sed (you must leve) we
wer scard and har stuck up we jumped and ran as
fat as we cud to are hows we lock op evreything
we luck out my windo we saw frankinstim and
gracla and his suns and monsers we cut not go to
sleep that nitght in the morning we went back to
the hontid hows we went in side a blob cot
Mickael gost wer in the Hall they did not see us
the door slamd We wir trapt the gosts flow at us
I ran. They toke Michael I saw war all the
stolen mony. The blob wos Josh and the fore
gosts wer Lowis wos the sciny gost. Branden wos
the fat gost. Grag wos the tall gost Kris wos
the small gost all of them came at me and old
Most West Winb came She scard the gosts and blob
awy I thank her. (She was my mother) we gote
Mickael he had a cut

Translation:

Me and Michael were walking down the long little path. It was raining, almost the middle of the night. We were coming home from a party. Along came Jimmy the Skunk. He said there was a haunted house down the road. We went to see. The rain was beating against the old, old house. The wind howled through the broken windows. A flash lit up the rooms. We saw bats. Then we heard thunder and the sound of footsteps on the stairs. We did not dare to look. And someone said, "You must leave." We were scared and our hair stuck up. We jumped and ran as fast as we could to our house. We locked up everything. We looked out my window. We saw Frankenstein and Dracula and his sons and monsters. We could not go to sleep that night. In the morning we went back to the haunted house. We went inside. A blob caught Michael. Ghosts were in the hall. They did not see us. The door slammed. We were trapped. The ghosts flew at us. I ran. They took Michael. I saw where all the stolen money (was). The blob was Josh and the four ghosts were Lewis, who was the skinny ghost; Branden, who was the fat ghost; Greg was the tall ghost; Kris was the small ghost. All of them came at me and Old Mother West Wind came. She scared the ghosts and blob away. I thanked her. (She was my mother.) We got Michael. He had a cut.

Commentary

Four major issues which surface frequently throughout Eli's story

I. The Issue of Attention

Attention is a complex system of brain controls that allows us to energize and regulate our thinking in our daily activities according to Mel Levine[1]. He compares the function of the attentional system to the role of the conductor of an orchestra. The conductor does not actually create the sounds of music. He controls the players of the instruments who in turn generate the actual melodies. In this analogy, attention serves as the conductor while the musicians are represented by the individual brain processes that are essential for learning, for behaving, and for relating well to other people.

Throughout his school years, several psychologists and pediatricians wondered if Eli had the condition termed 'Attention Deficit Dysfunction'. All testing and medication trials indicated the answer to be "no." However, using Levine's terminology, Eli has weak mental energy control. It is sometimes difficult for him to 'start up' his mental energy; once started, it is quickly used up. His mind is often 'over-active' as he tries to think through a thought, a problem, or a situation. Each thought triggers another tangent. This makes it seem like he is very distractible. However, Levine[2] states, "Distractibility is certainly not all bad. Distracted children are often very creative and insightful. They notice things others would miss or ignore. They are frequently described by their parents as incredibly observant. They perceive relationships between things that their more focused peers would never think of." This leads to great problem solving skill.

Eli

This description of distractibility indubitably applies to Eli. He is indeed very creative and quite insightful regarding other people. He certainly notices amazing things in the environment that many other people ignore. He is so observant that it often takes him longer to perform simple tasks, such as taking a walk, analyzing his food before eating, or, in school, thinking of what to write. What he needs are specific structures and memory hooks to help him stay on target.

Strategies that have been helpful to Eli as a young student in school

1. Provide goals or target points that he must achieve before he can move to another, more desired activity. For example in the chapter, *Homework*, Eli reports his 'rule' of not being able to play on his computer until he finishes his homework.

2. Provide reminders and triggers to help him stay on target. These offer a memory hook: it is a key that then triggers what he needs to remember. Examples include:
- The sign provided in the Homework chapter: *Eli: do the hardest first!*
- The mind map strategy reported in the Prequel. This strategy helps Eli focus on chunking and encourages him to think about doing a task, one step at a time.

A mind map is a diagram used to represent words, ideas, tasks or other items linked to and arranged around a central idea or word. It generates, visualizes, structures, and classifies ideas. It may be used as an aid in study, organization, problem-solving, decision writing, and organizing for pre-writing. It helps the student in visualizing the entire process or concept: it's essential to know where an idea comes from and where it's going.

The benefit of using a graphic organizer such as a mind map, semantic network or cognitive map, is that it is an image-centered diagram that represents semantic or other connections between portions of information. It is great for students like Eli who prefer images rather than words. It helps them analyze and concretely represent similarities and differences between two or three concepts or words. It is a valuable tool for developing comparing/contracting skills, which are critical prerequisite to inferential thinking. Furthermore, it encourages intuitive thinking because students first arrange the elements in a brain-storming manner, and then they can reorganize the items by importance. The Mid-Continent Regional Educational Laboratory has reported the graphic organizer to be the instructional technique with the greatest impact on information processing.

A few of the many valuable references that include samples of a variety of graphic organizer types include:

Online:
www.edHelper.com
www.smartdraw.com
www.inspirations.com
www.imindmap.com

Books:
LEARN: Playful Strategies for All Students[3]
The Source For Learning and Memory Strategies[4]
The Source For Reading Comprehension Strategies[5]

Eli

II. The Issue of Language

Efficient use of language is related to output or production, and includes both verbal language and written language. Successful output perpetuates motivation, feelings of overall effectiveness, and stable self-esteem. In contrast, when the output is inappropriate or inefficient, it becomes a source of "gnawing humiliation".[6] According to Levine, language production is one of the four forms of output. The other three are, motor production, organizational behavior, and problem solving.

Language production involves the process of converting ideas into spoken words. In school, this process needs to occur with tremendous speed, accuracy, and efficiency. Eli's language production issues are obvious in his 'low ideational density'. It takes a long time for him to say relatively little, especially when he is working with cognitive topics. He lacks cohesive ties and struggles to connect sentences together well. It's not that he doesn't have the ideas: his struggle involves putting his ideas into a language format. He strains to organize what he wants to say and is unable to expound upon his ideas because of these inefficiencies in organizing his thoughts while also using language. Consequently, he tends to use a non-elaborative style when speaking or writing, and writing conclusions presents a tremendous struggle.

Eli's problems with dysnomia further compound his efforts. For Eli, as with many students, these problems affect school language much more than social language. However, in some situations, Eli has trouble when speaking with his peers. This contributes to his quiet and shy mannerisms.

Dysnomia is a language production inefficiency, which varies significantly in degree, depending on the situation. It involves inadequacy in retrieving a specific word from memory at the moment it is needed. Many people occasionally experience a 'tip of the tongue' experience, wherein they struggle to recall a word or a name and feel that it is 'on the tip of their tongue'. However, individuals with dysnomia experience this situation much more frequently, and it often affects students in test taking situations, which is particularly frustrating.

The Boy Who Hated to Write

Eli deals with his dysnomia by referring to his teacher and his principal with labels, rather than by using their actual name, i.e., "Teacher" for his teacher's name. This avoids the embarrassment of forgetting the person's name. Throughout school, and continuing thereafter, he has struggled with recalling specific labels, titles, and especially people's names. In contrast, when Eli develops close ties with a person, he is able to more readily recall their name. This is why, in the Prequel, he refers to some by their names (Michael, Sam, Tammy) and others he refers to by their title (Teacher, Principal).

Another common habit Eli exhibited throughout school, related to his language production issues, involves his tendency for 'dumbing down' of thoughts. He expresses his ideas in simple language. While he is quite capable of thinking in a sophisticated manner, he finds it too demanding to translate complicated thoughts into verbal or written expression.

Strategies that have been helpful to Eli

1. Provide a memory hook or initiate opportunities for him to practice a name or specific word by clapping, using rhythm, or singing a tune with the name
2. Encourage elaboration by periodically reminding him how important it is to "build up his elaboration muscles"
3. Avoid embarrassing him: structure questions concretely when he is with his friends
4. Become a good listener and reward his language usage
5. Discourage the use of words such as "stuff" and "thing" and encourage him to become more specific
6. Provide speech and language therapy: Eli received language therapy from a licensed speech and language therapist for a few years during elementary school
7. Communicate to teachers the nature and extent of his struggles in this area
8. Provide concrete structure for activities that will require language usage, such as mind maps for writing, drawing a picture before describing an idea, closing eyes to visualize or imagine a scene before describing

Other specific recommendations that may be useful for all students who struggle with automatic rapid word retrieval include the following[7]:

- Keep notes handy for quick and easy reference
- Continue to develop strong vocabulary skills for more efficient word substitutions
- Develop vocabulary mnemonics
- Develop summary charts and tables and keep these readily accessible for quick access to information
- Use separate and clearly labeled binders/folders for different topics
- When making a phone call, even when calling family members, have a note card readily available with the names of spouses, children, or other pertinent information
- Post an enlarged list of frequently used phone numbers near each phone and/or use phones with automatic dialing
- Use visual aids or charts when explaining information to others
- Increase their vocabulary so that forgotten words can be substituted by another (such as *auto* for *car*) and learn to describe the desired word
- Use humor to cover for a misused or forgotten word

III. The Issue of Magical Thinking

Typically, a child at about age three utilizes magical thinking. This thinking is not reality-based, and the child may have trouble distinguishing among what actually are feelings, thoughts, and actions. As children mature, they begin to distinguish between reality and imagination.

Children with learning issues may experience perceptual development struggles and frequently feel anxious, worthless, and insignificant. A typical defense mechanism for dealing with the inefficiencies caused by learning struggle may be to develop an imaginary friend or helper, thus using magical thinking. These children typically engage in imaginative play long after their peers have stopped doing so.[8]

Eli demonstrated magical thinking in his relationship with his gnome, Peanut, in a number of ways. First, Peanut helped Eli implement the strategy of 'self-talk' and helped him think of the positive attributions that were his. Because it was difficult for Eli to take 'ownership' of these characteristics, he assigned them to his gnome. Secondly, he used magical thinking to decide that he would be smarter if he added checkmarks in Teacher's book, resulting in harder books to read. Third, Eli magically thought that running away would solve his problem with classwork. Eli's imaginary friend and his use of magical thinking proved useful over and over again.

In the Chapter, *The Meeting*, the adults develop a solution of the 'Red Card Plan.' This was an appropriate reaction to Eli's attempt to run away. It was critical to help him recognize that running away from a problem is not the correct solution but instead, is a magical thinking approach to the problem. To help him deal more realistically with problem-solving, he was, first, helped to understand the problem by including him in the meeting. Secondly, he was involved with developing the solution to fix the problem. Even though the adults actually created the 'Red Card Plan,' Eli's inclusion in the process was critical. As time progressed and Eli's problems continued, Eli was encouraged to get help by having a tutor. Eli needed to understand that running away from problems just causes them to get worse, whereas dealing with a problem makes it possible to find a solution.

IV. The Issue of Demystification

Mel Levine, throughout his books (*Keeping A Head in School*[9], *Educational Care*[10], *Developmental Variations*[11]), emphasizes that children cannot work on their problems if they do not really understand them. They need a vocabulary to capture and describe what they are trying to work on. Therefore, he recommends demystification: the process through which adults talk to children about the nature of their learning problems with the goal of enhancing their understanding.

"We cannot emphasize enough the importance of children understanding themselves. When they are unable to perceive the casual relationship between their specific weaknesses and the problems they are experiencing when they attend school, they tend to fantasize about themselves. Unfortunately, their fantasies are most often far worse than the realities. They may believe that they are retarded, crazy, or just born to lose. Such attributions promote fatalistic feelings and a strong belief that effort does no good in school. In addition, when children feel pervasively defective, they're likely to suffer a serious loss of motivation.

"Demystification is a process which provides children with more accurate personal insight. Through open discussions with adults who are working with them, they put borders around their deficits and come to recognize that like everyone else they have strengths and weaknesses. Very importantly, they learn the vocabulary of their problems. It is exceedingly hard to work on something when one doesn't know the name for it! If a student is confused in class, it is far healthier for him to think, "there goes my spatial processing problem again" than it is to feel, "Boy, am I a dummy."[12]

Levine elaborates upon five steps for providing demystification and he provides sample demystification discussions for the processes of attention, misunderstanding, deficient output, delayed skill acquisition, poor adaptation and reduced remembering in *Educational Care*[13]. His five steps include:
1. Introduction
2. Discussion of strengths
3. Discussion of weaknesses
4. Induction of optimism
5. Alliance formation

A vital aspect of demystification is to identify and reinforce the strengths and beauty in each child and adolescent. Several years ago, Dr. Robert Brooks introduced the metaphor, 'islands of competence' after analyzing many students' negative self-comments. He felt their comments suggested the students to be drowning in an ocean of self-perceived inadequacy and he concluded that if an ocean of inadequacy exists, then there must also be islands of competence. He defined these islands as areas that have been or have the potential to be sources of pride and accomplishments. Throughout his writings, he emphasizes the critical need to help children and adults identify and reinforce these islands, with the goal of helping the islands become more dominant in the ocean of inadequacy.[14]

Strategies that have been helpful to Eli

Throughout the Prequel, main story, and Epilogue, Eli is continually encouraged to find his islands of competence. His gnome, Peanut, is a concrete, although imagined, representation of the search for the islands of competence. Eli uses Peanut, along with other self-talk strategies, to accentuate his need for understanding himself and for analyzing his strengths and his weaknesses. Additionally, his strategies help him focus on his areas of strength so he can use these strengths to deal with weaknesses and thus, to accomplish his schoolwork. Being cognizant of his strengths allowed Eli to also take risks, such as when he ventured to describe Peanut with his friends, and when he allowed Sam to see his room, which was his own special domain.

Being able to understand himself and his learning style is probably the key factor involved with Eli's overall success, in spite of many learning challenges. Language-based learning disabilities, including dyslexia and dysgraphia, are lifelong issues. It is critical that we help these students learn to cope with *their life* as well as the daily activities in school.

In Chapter 2, *The Meeting*, the 'Red Card Plan' was a tremendous demystification tool. It helped increase the sensitivity of the adults and environment to Eli's excessive frustration. At the same time, the plan increased Eli's general coping skills. Having the red card available was similar to a relief valve for him, providing a tremendous source of reassurance. In actuality, Eli never needed to use the red card. Merely having it available was sufficient.

Dr. Brooks in *Raising Resilient Children*[14] offers a discussion of "Obstacles to Nurturing Islands of Competence" as well as "Principles For Experiencing Acceptance And Success." These lists include the following items.

Obstacles to Nurturing Islands of Competence[15]

1. The inability to experience the joy of success
2. Reinforcing low self-esteem
   Children often attribute whatever success they do attain to luck, chance, or fate. This reduces their confidence that they will be able to succeed in the future.

3. Misattributing success
   Children may choose negative activities as their goals for experiencing success, as for example becoming the class clown or engaging in antisocial activities.
4. Setting the bar too high
   Setting goals beyond what is realistic.
5. Parents defining a successful experience, from their own perspective
   This occurs when parents fail to recognize a child's great interest in an event or major issues of creativity, and instead only praise a sibling's academic competence.

In working with our students, it is essential to be realistic and to avoid obstacles to success, such as those identified by Brooks. We need to monitor our student's attributions as well as the reality of the established goals. As we do so, we need to be cognizant of our perspective in relationship to the child and his performances.

Principles for Experiencing Acceptance and Success[16]

1. Openly enjoy and celebrate child's accomplishments
2. Emphasize child's input in creating success
3. Identify and reinforce your child's islands of competence by engaging in environmental engineering
   This involves the creation of opportunities for the child to experience competence, as for example, providing Eli the opportunity to be "mechanical engineer" for the assembly equipment rather than engaging in oral reading in the classroom, or allowing him to tutor a kindergarten child, which gave him a positive role involving academics.
4. Gives strengths time to develop
   Children require time to develop and mature and it is critical for the relevant adults to be aware of this for each child. Eli was continually reinforced for his mechanical and creativity skills.
5. Accept unique strengths and successes of each child
   Children need to be accepted for who they are and not what we wish them to be. Children are aware of adult's disappointments when they don't meet perceived expectations and they are particularly sensitive when their successes are

not viewed as important or relevant by the important adults in their environment.

Above all, Brooks reminds us that *success is worth repeating.* It is critical for us to focus on the child's accomplishments as well as arrange opportunities for the child to succeed. These arrangements may involve manipulation of the task, the environment, and/or reactions of the adults.

In the Piano story of the Prequel, Eli reminisces about how something that begins very bad often turns into something good. This relates to the common saying, "when given a lemon, make lemonade." Throughout his school years, the message given him was to look for something good in a situation, even when it may begin in a negative way. As he grew older, the message included how to be proactive in turning negative situations into something more positive. For example, in high school he had a class where he experienced great difficulty completing the tests on time. He initiated a discussion with this teacher, which eventually solved the problem: he came to class early and began work on the first portion or question, thus allowing him the extra time.

Some recommendations for students, such as Eli, who become frustrated due to the need for extra effort, the difficulty of the task, and/or the multiple subparts of the tasks are as follows:[17]

1. Provide structure and coaching as necessary but also back off as much as possible to allow child to do the work
2. Set reasonable goals for the student and reasonable expectations for parents
3. Provide honest and specific reinforcements, as for example, "it is great that you did X"
4. Let the child know he is capable, using specific examples to emphasize that the task was difficult, the child did a great job, etc.
5. Focus on the child's strengths and affinities
6. Teach the child to accept compliments
7. Allow the child to experience some frustration, as tolerance of frustration is a necessary skill
8. Allow for mistakes: children learn from their mistakes and mistakes can be used as an opportunity for further growth
9. Help the child develop independence
10. Teach the child to be an effective self-advocate: this requires an understanding of the strengths as well as areas of struggle

Eli

Cerebrodiversity

Dr. Gordon Sherman coined the term *cerebrodiversity,* and it is one which incorporates many of the themes throughout this book. Dr. Sherman was formerly president of the International Dyslexia Association and assistant professor of neurology at Harvard Medical School, and once directed the Dyslexia Research Laboratory at Beth Israel Deaconess Medical Center in Boston. Currently a neuroscientist and school administrator, he is the author of more than 80 scientific articles, reviews, and books on learning differences.

Dr. Sherman states that we all have different brains. Every one of our brains is different and processes information differently. This variation is *cerebro*(brain)*diversity,* the cause of learning differences. It may result in some students having difficulties in the classroom, because there is no such thing as an ideal, optimal brain. Understanding that each individual processes information differently is the key to understanding basic learning differences. Sherman stresses that learning differences are not disabilities. "It is one's learning environment that makes learning differences problematic."

In his writings and conference presentations, Sherman emphasizes that dyslexia is a brain-based difference in processing information that affects a person's ability to read, write, and spell. Research has proven multiple times throughout the years that there is a real difference in the brains of those with dyslexia. Sherman always stresses that while dyslexia is often viewed as a disability, many times those with dyslexia have a distinct talent, such as mechanical aptitude, a creative approach to problem-solving, visualization, artistic expression, or athletic ability.

This concept of having all kinds of minds and cerebrodiversity is a constant theme throughout Eli's stories as he discusses his struggles, his strengths, and in his conclusions about issues. It is critical for all children who experience struggle with learning to have at least a basic understanding of these concepts. Eli emphasized this concept when, in college, he wrote his allegory about the Eagles (Epilogue).

Commentary on other issues appearing within Eli's story

Compensatory Techniques

1. Compensations

Eli uses compensations throughout his school tasks, especially for writing. Being able to use the computer was critical for him for two reasons:
1. It helped relieve the hand fatigue caused by manipulating a pencil.
2. It identified misspelled words. While he still must be careful regarding homonyms and other words substitutions, the computer enabled him to recognize most of his misspelled words and correct them as needed with the Franklin[18], as discussed in Chapter 1. Once able to use the computer automatically, Eli was able to expend his cognitive energy on the process of writing: separating out extraneous thoughts and integrating the multiple processes necessary.

It was essential to teach Eli computer skills using strategies that differed from most conventional classroom teaching. His computer program included dual goals.

- The first goal was basic keyboarding. He practiced keyboarding using typing tutor programs every day for a specified number of minutes, using a timer. Initially, he practiced only for 5 minutes a day, but his practice increased to about 15 minutes daily, as he grew older. He was to attend fully, not look at the keyboard, and use correct fingering while he practiced.
- The second goal involved using the computer to compose sentences. When thinking about content, he did not focus on correct fingering.

Eli's focus was to be solely on the content until such time his keyboard fingering became completely automatic. As a young teen, he joined a young teen internet group and by 9th grade, he was typing 65 words per minute, with mostly correct fingering. It was apparent that his dual goal program was a success.

Separating these processes while learning to type is critical for many LD students who experience struggles with typical keyboard programs. The main reasons for their struggles include having to stay at the keyboard for too long without breaks, the pressures on attaining speed, and overload caused by having to focus simultaneously on fingering and content before reaching automaticity.

The Franklin Language Master 6000b[18] was extremely helpful for Eli in correcting his misspelled words, primarily because of its speaking component, which allowed him to type in the word phonetically and then obtain a list of possibilities. He could listen to each word in the list and then select the word he desired. Having this auditory input was critical in the process and helped him develop greater skill (Chapters 1 and 5).

In elementary school, Eli only imagined being able to talk to his computer and have it type on its own. This became a reality for him in college as he established skill in using voice-activated word processing, such as *Dragon Naturally Speaking[19]*. (Epilogue).

Another compensation for Eli was the development of the 'Red Card Plan' (Chapter 2). This helped Eli deal with his feelings of extreme frustration and helped to adjust the environment more favorably for him.

2. Self-talk

The use of self-talk was an extremely valuable strategy for Eli throughout his school years, and it continues to be an important strategy in his adult life. Eli used self-talk with his animals while in his fort, as well as in his 'interactions' with Peanut. Self-talk can be aloud, as with younger students, or silently when more socially appropriate.

Self-talk can be a mental preparation strategy whereby students talk to themselves in an attempt to enhance their self-confidence, remember sequences or information, or focus on affirmations. Using self-talk can help refocus concentration, especially when paying attention to positives rather than negatives.

This strategy was discussed in 1934 by Vygotsky, who stresses that child development is the result of interactions between people and and their social environment, including written language. The child, through interactions, develops higher mental functions and complex mental processes that are intentional, self-regulated, and mediated by language and other sign systems. Examples of these higher mental functions include focused attention, deliberate memory, and formal verbal thinking. One of the best-known concepts illustrating Vygotsky's view of language is that of private speech or self-talk: speech directed to oneself. (Lev Semenovich Vygotsky, *Thought and Language*).

3. Creativity

Eli demonstrates a great deal of creativity through his imaginations, spatial constructions, and in his interactions with his friends. In second grade, his stories were much more creative and thoughtful, as expressed in Chapter 1. It is a definite shame that his stories decreased in creativity because of the stress of the multiple components needed for efficient writing and his difficulties with his working memory.

Related to Eli's high level of creativity is his superb visual thinking. West defines visual thinking as that "form of thought in which images are generated or recalled in the mind and are manipulated, overlaid, translated, associated with other similar forms (as with a metaphor), rotated, increased or reduced in size, distorted, or otherwise transformed gradually from one familiar image to another. These images may be visual representations of material things or they may be nonphysical, abstract concepts manipulated in the same way as visual forms".[20] It is related to spatial ability and pattern recognition.

Pattern recognition is exceptionally strong for Eli and is defined by West as "the ability to discern similarities of form among two or more things, whether these be tactile designs, facial resemblance of family members, graphs of repeating biological growth cycles, or similarities between historical epochs". Pattern recognition is related to problem-solving in its involvement of the recognition of a developing or repeating pattern and the carrying out of actions to obtain desired results based on one's understanding of this pattern. Problem-solving may also be considered nearly synonymous with some of the most important forms of creativity.[21]

Instructional Strategies

1. Structured Multisensory Instruction

Traditional instructional programs are usually less appropriate for students with dyslexia, because these students do not process language the same way as others. This is why Eli progressed so much more efficiently once he began to work individually with his teacher and later with a tutor: the one-on-one instruction was the critical factor for him, especially because they followed the philosophy of "if he doesn't learn the way we teach, we'll teach the way he learns." In other words, they used diagnostic teaching and adjusted their methods to his progress and understanding. This strategy, combined with the use of structured multisensory instruction, was the winning combination for Eli.

Dyslexic students specifically need instruction that is clear, organized, and multisensory. These students are often good thinkers, but they need help to understand how to go about the task. The best teaching approach focuses on the interrelationships between reading, spelling, and writing using structured language and a special type of phonics program that includes phonological training. They need to understand how letters represent speech, that sounds are blended to make words, and that long words can be divided into smaller parts or syllables. They must also learn the rules and generalizations governing English. Writing must integrate motor skills, punctuation, grammar, spelling, usage, and organization and sequencing of thoughts.

Multisensory teaching should include seeing (working with print), listening, and feeling and doing. Active participation in learning is critical to help students to focus their attention and to remember. Because students with dyslexia forget easily, instruction needs to include constant review, until they know it to a mastery level, and then occasional review thereafter. Furthermore, it is critical for success to be the goal of every lesson, enabling students to feel that they have achieved their best.

Multisensory Structured Language Teaching includes these components:

- Simultaneous multisensory teaching: teaching is simultaneously visual, auditory, and kinesthetic/tactile in order to enhance learning and memory. When students with dyslexia use several senses at the same time, clinical evidence demonstrates that they are better able to store the necessary language information in their brains. The multisensory strategies help focus attention on what they are learning.
- Direct instruction: teachers directly explain and demonstrate all skills and concepts to students with continuous student-teacher interaction. Inferential learning of any concept is not taken for granted.
- Systematic and cumulative instruction: teachers present reading and writing skills sequentially and cumulatively. Whenever students learn a new concept, they must integrate it with concepts already mastered. Instruction must follow the logical order of the language, beginning with the easiest and most basic elements and progressing systematically to more difficult levels. Students must have opportunity for ample and extended practice as well as systematic review.
- Diagnostic teaching: teachers base the teaching plan on careful and continuous assessment of the student's needs.
- Analytic and synthetic instruction: teaching linguistic principles must be both whole-to-part (analysis) and part-to-whole (synthesis). The teacher works in both directions for all concepts, whether the student is learning to encode or decode words, or at a more complicated level, to put words together to write a meaningful sentence or to pull them apart for comprehension.

2. Visual organizers

Effective writing is absolutely dependent on good organization skills, and this aspect is critical for students who learn differently. Generally, students who struggle to sort and organize language–based information will also struggle with clarity, conciseness, and effectiveness of written assignments. It is imperative that such students understand how to structure different tasks for different purposes. Concrete visual techniques are extremely helpful and include a wide range of strategies such as pre-writing worksheets, frames, visual organizers, mind maps, and clusters.

Organization should be very thorough, specific, and well taught. It may, in essence, be the most critical aspect of the writing process for the dyslexic and dysgraphic student, as it was for Eli. It is crucial to address the organizational deficits so commonly found in these students.

Visual organization strategies are effective, because they provide a concrete alternative to traditional outlining. This allows students to organize material in a visual pattern which enables them to see the relationships among the information. It facilitates their ability to represent connections more easily while promoting fluency, flexibility, and more originality.

As Eli describes in the Prequel, having a checklist of the steps to use when writing is imperative. In this example, he used a very simplistic visual organizer that contained one larger circle for the main idea and three circles for supporting facts. Having this framework (the basic form of a circle for main idea and smaller circles for supporting facts) helped him focus on the main components of his writing assignment, highlighting one portion at a time. As he progressed through the grades, he learned how to use and select from a wide range of other visual organizers appropriate for a specific task.

Memory Stategies

Mnemonics, such as acrostics, acronyms, and key words, are essential for some students because their ability to conceptualize is much stronger than their semantic memory, or recall of specific words. Using mnemonics with great frequency was a critical component contributing to Eli's academic successes.

Some of the many specific strategy examples include the following.

The Boy Who Hated to Write

Acrostic phrases or sentences: the first letter of each word represents what you are trying to remember. These may be silly sentences or a phrase, as in these examples:

- *Every good boy does fine* to remember the names of notes in music

- *Roy G. Biv* to recall the sequence of the colors of the rainbow: red, orange, yellow, green, blue, indigo, violet

- *Dear Ms. Sally Brown* to remember the steps for long division (divide, multiply, subtract, bring down)

Acronyms: a single word is made from the first letter of each bit of information you need to remember. Some examples include these:

- *HOMES* to remember the names of the Great Lakes (Huron, Ontario, Michigan, Erie, and Superior)

- *FACE* to recall the notes within spaces on a musical staff

- *TAG* and *FIRE* to recall the two major alliance groups: countries in the Central Powers (Turkey, Austria-Hungry, Germany) and countries in the Allied Powers (France, Italy, Russia, England)

Graphics, other visual formats, and visualizations are useful tools to trigger memory. In the Prequel, Eli describes using a picture of a Brachiosaurus. In Chapter 1, Eli's mom had given him a sign to remind him to "Do the hardest 1st". In Chapter 3, Eli uses visual spatial strategies to help find his way out of the cave.

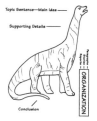

Key words: a familiar word, visualization, and/or gesture can help associate the key information with the word you're trying to remember. It is helpful to make these associations humorous, and even absurd, although meaningful, as in these examples:

- Learning the vocabulary term "biome" by remembering "a biome is a <u>home</u> for animals"

- Saying the phrase, "hippocampus chomp, chomp" while moving your hands in a chomping motion to help recall that the hippocampus feature of the brain helps us grab information to increase our memory

- Learning a specific key word to help remember a given sound-symbol relationship, such as, a-apple, t-tiny, m-monkeys, k-kiss

This strategy is even more intensive when organizing two or more keywords into a phrase and associated illustration, such as, *"tiny monkeys kiss fat pigs"* (MFR[22])

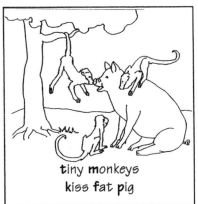

tiny monkeys
kiss fat pig

Visual Menmonic picture clue for letters
t, m, k, f, p
Memory Foundations for Reading [22]

Repetition and rehearsal: the more you rehearse information, the more efficiently facts are stored in memory. Rehearsing information using one or more of the mnemonic strategies provides a "hook." Incorporating categorization enhances the recall potential of information. Further enhance your memory rehearsal strategies by simultaneously incorporating any of these components:

- Rhyme
- Rhythm
- Gestures
- Humor
- Visuals, including color

Following is a mnemonic story about Eli learning state capitals[23].

The Boy Who Hated to Write

One day in fifth grade, Eli came home from school upset because he had to learn the state capitals. I was at first confused because he had been learning individual state capitals and other facts (such as, state bird) for several years. Associative memory for some rote material was difficult for him, but with perseverance and substantial multisensory practice, he was usually successful — at least for the short-term. This situation was different because he had to learn all 50 state capitals at once.

To help ease his panic, we first made a list of the various rehearsal strategies he could use. His list included the following strategies:

- Chunking: he would work on only one state capital at a time
- Spiraling: each time he finished with one state, he would review all the states he had learned so far
- Downtime: he would study in small chunks of time, allowing himself plenty of downtime between sessions
- Recognition before retrieval:
- He typed the name of each State on a blue index card and he typed the name of each capital onto yellow index card
- He typed an alphabetical list of all the states, along with their capital, to use for reference
- He studied each state and its capital in two ways (this is the recognition strategy):
    - He looked at the blue card with the state name and then selected, from three or four choices, the appropriate capital (yellow cards)
    - He looked at the yellow card with the capital and then selected, from three or four choices, the appropriate state name (blue cards)
- He tested his knowledge of the match using traditional flash card methods (this is the retrieval strategy):
    - Looking at the state's name on a blue card, he said the capital
    - Looking at the capital on a yellow card, he said the state name
- Each time he confirmed his response, either with an assistant or with his reference sheet

Eli

- Mnemonics: he used pictured mnemonics for difficult state names, using the Bornstein mnemonics cards[24]
- Movement activities: he devised a number of activities that incorporated saying the states in capitals while jumping on a tramp (mini-trampoline or exerciser)
- Goal setting: he determined, using a calendar, how much time he had before the test date and he set goals for:
  Knowing 10 capitals
  Knowing 20 capitals
  Knowing 30 capitals
  Knowing 40 capitals
  Knowing all 50 capitals

Having this list and action plan helped relieve Eli's sense of panic and his feeling of being overwhelmed. He began to feel more comfortable that with enough effort, he could achieve his goal of being successful on this test. He was right and he triumphed, receiving an A+ on his test.

The irony of this story is that Eli's teacher was quite used to his poor spelling and accommodated this issue, which is a good thing. However, I was aware that some of his "misspellings" on this test were actually confusions with the mnemonics used: he remembered the mnemonic, but couldn't quite remember the word it stood for. For example, he studied a picture of a guy named *Cal* who had a sack of memos. The sack of memos was to remind him of *Sacramento* and *Cal* was a cue for the state's name, *California*. On his test, next to the word *California*, Eli wrote *Sakememo*.

Was this an actual spelling error?

Was it poor associative retrieval of the pair of words?

Did Eli need additional practice in the actual words that the mnemonic was to cue?

We still aren't sure which of these, or which combination, provides the actual answer to his struggle. When teaching mnemonics to students, it is the essential to ensure that they have enough practice with the actual words or phrase represented by the mnemonic.

One of the most valuable concepts for teachers and parents regarding the issue of students struggling with memory is summarized in this quote, "Your students may not remember what you taught them, but they will remember how you made them feel." (Anonymous)

Teacher Understanding

Enabling a student to develop the resilience and motivation needed to continue a difficult task can be a challenge. To help accomplish this, the teacher or parent must communicate a positive perspective and express a real understanding of the student's efforts towards the final product. Examples include Eli's teacher's positive comments about his crafts in the Prequel and the principal's observation of Eli's distress in Chapter 2. Conversely, negative comments may generate often extremely negative and destructive reactions, as in Chapter 3.

To help a teacher develop greater perspective regarding the dyslexic and dysgraphic student, and his unexpected and exaggerated strengths and weaknesses, Michael Ryan[25] responded to the question, "Why does the dyslexic child have extreme ups and downs?" He states, "Inconsistencies in performance plague the dyslexic child. The fact that he cannot rely on his memory for symbols in words can produce havoc in his life. Although everyone has strong and weak points, and everyone has ups and downs, the child with dyslexia may have unexpected and exaggerated strengths and weaknesses. For example, the student may be extremely good in the logic of mathematics but not be able to remember a telephone number. The student may be a natural leader of others but not be able to remember the names of people she meets. The student may be great at drawing objects but not be able to spell the simplest words such as "of," "they," or "said."

"These inconsistencies produce a "roller coaster" effect. At times, the dyslexic students can perform far better than the abilities of his or her peers. At times, however, he or she may not accomplish the simplest tasks correctly. Many adults with dyslexia compare this to "walking into black holes". Dyslexic students benefit from a thorough understanding of the symptoms to help them anticipate the conditions under which they are most likely to succeed.

"The dyslexic student may also perform unevenly within tasks. That is, even the errors may be inconsistent. In a 100-word essay, the student may misspell the same word three different times and three different ways. In one sentence, the student may recognize the word and misread it in the next. This type of variability is frustrating and difficult for everyone to understand and accept.

"Finally, the performance of the dyslexic student may vary from day to day. On some days, reading may be fairly easy. Yet on another day, he may barely be able to write his name. This inconsistency is extremely confusing, not only to the student, but to everyone else.

"In comparison, few handicapping conditions are intermittent".

In a study from Columbia University, 800 adolescents with learning problems identified the most frustrating aspect of their learning disability. The majority of students cited performance inconsistency, stating, "The problem seems to come and go. I never know from one day to the next how I will perform in school." This is indeed frustrating.[26]

Lavoie states that a major teacher strategy for increasing students' motivation is to establish and maintain appropriate relationships with students. He offers a large number of suggestions of "small but insignificant things that a teacher can do or say to build an effective working relationship with students." Some examples include:
- Make eye contact with students when they speak
- Listen closely to them and use body language to let them know you're interested in what they're telling you
- Use their names often in conversations and discussions and include their names in written corrections
- Avoid sarcasm
- Communicate your confidence by assuming success, not failure
- Never, *ever*, express disappointment in a child

- Provide students with several ways to demonstrate their skills and knowledge

Dyslexia

Dyslexia is a reading and language disorder that is a lifelong condition. Children with dyslexia have difficulty with reading, spelling, writing, and related language skills that is unexpected in relation to intelligence and educational opportunity. The individual's ability to understand, analyze, and use systems of language is inefficient.

Dyslexia is a lifelong, intrinsic condition that is modified by instruction. The manifestations of dyslexia change as the individual grows and learns, although the underlying causal factors tend to be stable. What begins as a problem with speech sound awareness, letter recognition, or verbal expression becomes a problem with sounding out new written words, acquiring a site vocabulary, recalling basic spellings, and producing written compositions. The disorder in older students often causes slow and inaccurate reading, poor spelling, disorganized writing, and difficulty with learning foreign languages.

The core of dyslexia is the phonological deficit. When learning to read, the students have trouble identifying the separate speech sounds that make up words (phonemes) or the letters (graphemes) that represent these speech sounds. These phonemic or phonological difficulties cause struggles in reading words out of context, pronouncing new words, distinguishing similar words, placing or identifying accent, or remembering visual or verbal information. These core struggles are often associated with selected difficulties in comprehension and written expression.

Dysgraphia

Dysgraphia is defined as a difficulty in automatically remembering and mastering the sequence of muscle motor movements needed in writing letters or numbers. This difficulty is out of harmony with the person's intelligence, regular teaching instruction, and (in most cases) the use of the pencil in non-learning tasks. It is neurologically based and exists in varying degrees, ranging from mild to moderate. It can be diagnosed, and it can be overcome if appropriate remedial strategies are taught well and conscientiously carried out. An adequate remedial program generally works if applied on a daily basis. In many situations, it is relatively easy to plan appropriate compensations to be used as needed.

Dysgraphia is an inefficiency, which seldom exists without other symptoms of learning problems. While it may occasionally exist alone, it is most commonly related to learning problems involved within the sphere of written language. Difficulty in writing is often a major problem for students, especially as they progress into upper elementary and into secondary school. Rosa Hagan, in an address to IDA, has stated, "Inefficiency in handwriting skills provides a barrier to learning, whereas efficiency in basic handwriting skills provides a tool for learning. Once this tool is established, it can help reinforce many other areas kids are having difficulties with."

Many students with dyslexia may also experience writing struggles. Dysgraphia differs from dyslexia in several important processing components; however, the strategies for remediation and compensations are identical, regardless of the etiology. Many students may struggle with both dyslexia and dysgraphia, as is the case with Eli.

In 1998, Melvin D. Levine wrote a Foreword to *The Writing Dilemma*[27]. Portions are included below.

What's Riding on Writing

"Why place a high premium on the writing abilities of students? After all, there are surprisingly few careers that necessitate exemplary expository or creative writing skills. Nor is success in the adult world predicated upon accurate spelling, an adaptive pencil grasp, or aesthetically impressive legibility. In fact, when you grow up, you are at liberty to write in either cursive or manuscript, rely on a computer or dictating machine, overutilize a spellchecker, or conveniently confine your paper trail repertory to filling out forms and writing checks (although credit cards have diminished the need even for the latter graphomotor subscale). Perhaps, therefore, it is time for children to be granted once and for all the right not to write!

The Boy Who Hated to Write

Having assumed the role of devil's advocate and drastically trivialized the act, I will state my case for writing and support the laudable mission of the current unique monograph, *The Writing Dilemma*. Writing indeed represents the ultimate neurocognitive integrative act. It is a supreme accomplishment of the developing on mind. It is in the act of writing, and only in the act of writing, that a seemingly diverse collection of germinating neurodevelopmental functions and academic subskills coalesce and collaborate. Writing demands the vigorous participation of attention, multiple forms of memory, language, critical and creative thought, brainstorming, motor output, metacognition, progressive automization, organization, synchronization, and even visualization. In addition, writing represents a formidable challenge to problem solving skill, as exigencies, such as planning, previewing, topic selection, strategy use, self-monitoring, and pacing represent core components of the problem solving act. Writing is as well a social skill, as renditions on paper are cautiously guided by the author's conscious insights into the backgrounds, preferences, and expectations of prospective readers (including the ever-changing parade of requirements and personal tastes found among individual teachers).

Too obvious inferences can be drawn: first of all, writing is a wide-open window on central nervous system development and function. This is especially the case during the middle childhood years, ages 10 to 15, when writing facility or difficulty is a commentary on the ways in which critical neurodevelopmental functions are progressing and becoming tightly interwoven. Second, it should be obvious that in the process of becoming a writer, a student is honing and blending the widest possible range of subskills and underlying brain processes. Thus, writing serves to solidify and integrate the very same functions that are needed to master writing in the first place! Regrettably, some students harbor neurodevelopmental dysfunctions or variations that thwart writing attainment. Some become writing phobic. They write as little and has passively as they can. As a result, these nonwriters lose ground with respect to language progression, memory capacity, organizational skill and other essential abilities that we have mentioned. While most careers do not stress writing, they all call for strengths in writing's neurocognitive underpinnings.

There exists a multitude of possible reasons (and very commonly combinations of reasons) for a student's writing failure or reluctance. Consequently, there are many subtypes of writing disorder. When we come to understand the reasons for a particular child's writing difficulty, we have learned an enormous amount about that individuals intrinsic 'wiring'. That which we have so discovered and uncovered can have vital implications for understanding the whole child, and for substantially heightening his or her level of academic productivity as well as pride.

Up until now, writing has been a well guarded territory narrowly divided between professional disciplines. When psycholinguistics or speech and language pathologists have spoken of written problems, they referred to them as disabilities of written language. Motor specialists have assumed that writing problems are the result of neuromuscular coordination deficits. Others have invoked exclusively attention deficits, laziness (and like forms of moral turpitude), performance anxiety, or other simplistic, global, and rather monopolistic attributions for all writing failure.

Clearly, it is time for holistic approach to the understanding of writing and of problems with writing.

No child needs or deserves to suffer writing humiliation, we assert penitently!"

Dr. Mel Levine

Professor of Pediatrics
University of North Carolina Medical School
Director, The Clinical Center for the Study of Development and Learning
Founding President, All Kinds of Minds, A Nonprofit Institute for the
Understanding of Differences in Learning

Footnotes

1 Levine, Melvin D. (2002). Educational Care, 2nd Edition, page 18. Massachusetts: Educators Publishing Service.

2 Levine (2002). Page 32

3 Richards, Regina G. (2001). LEARN: Playful Strategies for All Students. Riverside, CA: RET Center Press

4 Richards, Regina G. (2003). The Source for Learning and Memory Strategies. East Moline, Ill: Linguisystems, Inc.

5 Richards,m Regina G. (2006). The Source for Reading Comprehension Strategies. East Moline, Ill: Linguisystems, Inc.

6 Levine (2002). Page 142

7 Richards (2001). Page 33

8 Levine (2002). Page 134

9 Levine, Melvin D. (1990). Keeping A Head in School. East Moline, Ill: Linguisystems, Inc.

10 Levine (2002).

11 Levine, Melvin D. (1998). Developmental Variation and Learning Disorders, 2nd Edition. Massachusetts: Educators Publishing Service.

12 Levine (2002). Page 283

13 Levine (2002). Pages 283-285

14 Brooks, Robert and Goldstein, Sam (2001). Raising Resilient Children: Fostering Strength, Hope and Optimism in Your Child. Chicago, Ill: Contemporary Books

15 Brooks (2001). Pages 138-146

16 Brooks (2001). Pages 147-165

17 Richards (2001). Page 32

18 Franklin Language Master, www.franklin.com

19 Dragon Naturally Speaking, www.Nuance.com or www.dragontalk.com

20 West, Thomas G. (1997). In the Mind's Eye: Visual Thinkers, Gifted People with Dyslexia and Other Learning Difficulties, Computer Images and the Ironies of Creativity, page 21. Amherst, New York: Prometheus Books

21 West (1997). Page 22

22 Richards, Regina G. (1997). Memory Foundations for Reading: Visual Mnemonics for Sound/Symbol Relationships. Riverside, CA: RET Center Press

23 Richards (2003). Pages 191 and 192.

24 Bornstein, Arthur (1983). States and Capitals: Memorization System. West Los Angeles, CA: Bornstein School of Memory Training

25 Ryan, Michael (1994). The Other Sixteen Hours: The Social and Emotional Problems of Dyslexia. Baltimore, MD: The International Dyslexia Association

26 Lavoie, Richard (2007). The Motivation Breakthrough: 6 Secrets to Turning On The Tuned-Out Child, page 28. New York, New York: Simon & Schuster, Touchstone Books

27 Levine, Melvin D. (1998 – currently out of print). In Richards, Regina G. The Writing Dilemma: Understanding Dysgraphia. Riverside, CA: RET Center Press

AUTHOR INFORMATION

Eli I. Richards graduated in 2001 from DeVry Institutes with a bachelor of science degree in telecommunications management. His first job was at the Ontario Airport Information Management Division for a few years. Next, he worked at Electronic Arts (EA) for three years, which enabled him to be involved in the video game industry before he entered the network security field. He now works as a Senior Information Security Analyst at VISA, Inc. Eli's current hobbies are camping, hiking, video games, sports, bike riding, and computers.

Eli has been interested in computers since elementary school, when he helped teachers set up and operate their new computers. In middle school, he worked in the library, setting up the first multimedia computer system. As a junior, he established the first website for his

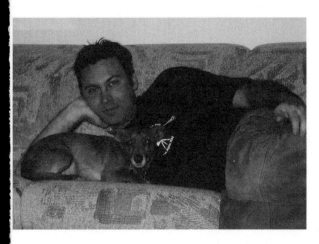

High School. At that time, he also initiated the website for the Inland Empire Branch of the International Dyslexia Association (www.dyslexia-ca.org), which he maintained for many years and for which he continues to provide consultant services. In 1995, Eli received the Student Volunteer Award from the Southern California Consortium of the International Dyslexia Association. When receiving the award Eli stated, "I like helping IDA because it helps teachers and parents understand kids who learn differently. One of the most important things a kid needs for success is to have teachers and parents who understand and encourage him."

Regina G. Richards, M.A., President of Richards Educational Therapy Center, is founder and former Director of Big Springs School and Ed Therapy Center. This Center specializes in multidisciplinary programs for language learning disabilities, especially dyslexia and dysgraphia. She began practicing as an Educational Therapist in Riverside in 1975, although she began her career in bilingual education, working on curriculum development and test design.

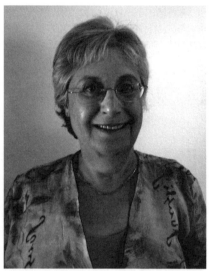

Regina has authored a variety of journal articles, articles on LD on Line (www.ldonline.org) and books on visual development, reading, dyslexia, dysgraphia, and memory. Her publications include the following from LinguiSystems (www.linguisystems.com): *The Source for Dyslexia and Dysgraphia, The Source for Learning and Memory*, and T*he Source for Reading Comprehension Strategies.* Other publications, available from RET Center Press (www.retctrpress.com), include: *LEARN: Playful Strategies for All Learners, Memory Foundations for Reading: Visual Mnemonics for Sound/symbol Assocation,* and *When Writing's a Problem.*

She has been very active in her local branch of the International Dyslexia Assocation and is currently President. She speaks at conferences and workshops nationally and frequently teaches at the University of California Extension programs in Riverside and in San Diego.